The **National Academy of Sciences** was established in 1863 by an Act of Congress, signed by President Lincoln, as a private, nongovernmental institution to advise the nation on issues related to science and technology. Members are elected by their peers for outstanding contributions to research. Dr. Marcia McNutt is president.

The **National Academy of Engineering** was established in 1964 under the charter of the National Academy of Sciences to bring the practices of engineering to advising the nation. Members are elected by their peers for extraordinary contributions to engineering. Dr. John L. Anderson is president.

The **National Academy of Medicine** (formerly the Institute of Medicine) was established in 1970 under the charter of the National Academy of Sciences to advise the nation on medical and health issues. Members are elected by their peers for distinguished contributions to medicine and health. Dr. Victor J. Daze is president.

The three Academies work together as the **National Academies of Sciences, Engineering, and Medicine** to provide independent, objective analysis and advice to the nation and conduct other activities to solve complex problems and inform public policy decisions. The National Academies also encourage education and research, recognize outstanding contributions to knowledge, and increase public understanding in matters of science, engineering, and medicine.

Learn more about the National Academies of Sciences, Engineering, and Medicine at **www.nationalacademies.org**.

Consensus Study Reports published by the National Academies of Sciences, Engineering, and Medicine document the evidence-based consensus on the study's statement of task by an authoring committee of experts. Reports typically include findings, conclusions, and recommendations based on information gathered by the committee and the committee's deliberations. Each report has been subjected to a rigorous and independent peer-review process and it represents the position of the National Academies on the statement of task.

Proceedings published by the National Academies of Sciences, Engineering, and Medicine chronicle the presentations and discussions at a workshop, symposium, or other event convened by the National Academies. The statements and opinions contained in proceedings are those of the participants and are not endorsed by other participants, the planning committee, or the National Academies.

Rapid Expert Consultations published by the National Academies of Sciences, Engineering, and Medicine are authored by subject-matter experts on narrowly focused topics that can be supported by a body of evidence. The discussions contained in rapid expert consultations are considered those of the authors and do not contain policy recommendations. Rapid expert consultations are reviewed by the institution before release.

For information about other products and activities of the National Academies, please visit www.nationalacademies.org/about/whatwedo.

COMMITTEE ON RISK ANALYSIS METHODS FOR NUCLEAR WAR AND NUCLEAR TERRORISM

WILLIAM C. OSTENDORFF, U.S. Navy (Retired), *Co-Chair*
M. ELISABETH PATÉ-CORNELL (NAE), Stanford University, *Co-Chair*
DAVID L. BANKS, Duke University
VICKI M. BIER, University of Wisconsin–Madison (Retired)
MATTHEW G. BUNN,[1] Harvard University
NANCY J. COOKE, Arizona State University
RAYMOND JEANLOZ (NAS), University of California, Berkeley
MADHAV V. MARATHE, University of Virginia
RICHARD W. MIES, The Mies Group, Ltd.
GREGORY S. PARNELL, University of Arkansas
SCOTT D. SAGAN, Stanford University
JAMES SCOURAS, Johns Hopkins University Applied Physics Laboratory
PAUL SLOVIC (NAS), Decision Research and University of Oregon
ALYSON G. WILSON, North Carolina State University

Staff

CARL-GUSTAV ANDERSON, Program Officer, Board on Mathematical Sciences and Analytics, *Co-Study Director* (until February 2022)
JENNY HEIMBERG, Senior Program Officer, Nuclear and Radiation Studies Board, *Co-Study Director*
MARGUERITE SCHNEIDER, Administrative Coordinator, Intelligence Community Studies Board
MICHELLE SCHWALBE, Director, Board on Mathematical Sciences and Analytics
CHARLES FERGUSON, Senior Board Director, Nuclear and Radiation Studies Board
BRITTANY SEGUNDO, Program Officer, Board on Mathematical Sciences and Analytics
MICAH LOWENTHAL, Director, Committee on International Security and Arms Control

[1] Resigned February 2022.

NUCLEAR AND RADIATION STUDIES BOARD

WILLIAM H. TOBEY, Los Alamos National Laboratory, *Chair*
JAMES A. BRINK, Massachusetts General Hospital, *Vice Chair*
SALLY A. AMUNDSON, Columbia University
STEVEN M. BECKER, Old Dominion University
AMY BERRINGTON DE GONZALEZ, National Cancer Institute
MADELYN R. CREEDON, Green Marble Group, LLC
SHAHEEN A. DEWJI, Georgia Institute of Technology
PAUL T. DICKMAN, Argonne National Laboratory
STEPAN KALMYKOV, Moscow State University
ALLISON M. MACFARLANE, University of British Columbia
ELEANOR MELAMED, National Nuclear Security Administration (Retired)
PER F. PETERSON (NAE), University of California, Berkeley
R. JULIAN PRESTON, Environmental Protection Agency
MONICA C. REGALBUTO, Idaho National Laboratory
HENRY D. ROYAL, Washington University in St. Louis

Staff

CHARLES FERGUSON, Director
LESLIE BEAUCHAMP, Program Assistant
DARLENE GROS, Senior Program Assistant
JENNY HEIMBERG, Senior Program Officer
MICHAEL JANICKE, Senior Program Officer
OURANIA KOSTI, Senior Program Officer
LAURA LLANOS, Financial Business Partner

COMMITTEE ON INTERNATIONAL SECURITY AND ARMS CONTROL

RAYMOND JEANLOZ (NAS), University of California, Berkeley, *Chair*
LINTON F. BROOKS, Independent Consultant
MATTHEW G. BUNN, Harvard University
STEVEN A. FETTER, University of Maryland
DAVID R. FRANZ, Kansas State University
RICHARD L. GARWIN (NAS/NAE/NAM), IBM Thomas J. Watson Research Center
ROSE E. GOTTEMOELLER, Stanford University
DIANE E. GRIFFIN (NAS/NAE), Johns Hopkins University
MARGARET E. HAMBURG (NAM), Nuclear Threat Initiative
MORIBA K. JAH, The University of Texas at Austin
ALASTAIR I. JOHNSTON, Harvard University
LORA LANNAN SAALMAN, Stockholm International Peace Research Institute
ROBERT H. LATIFF, R. Latiff Associates
JAMES W. LEDUC, Galveston National Laboratory
HERBERT S. LIN, Stanford University
DOUGLAS L. LOVERRO, Loverro Consulting, LLC
RICHARD A. MESERVE (NAE), Covington & Burling, LLP
RICHARD W. MIES, The Mies Group, Ltd.
PETER PALESE (NAS/NAM), The Mount Sinai Hospital
VICTORIA A. SAMSON, Secure World Foundation
JIM TIMBIE, Stanford University

JOHN G. HILDEBRAND (NAS), University of Arizona, *Ex Officio Member*

Staff

MICAH LOWENTHAL, Director
NICOLE CERVENKA, Research Associate
RITA GUENTHER, Senior Program Officer
HOPE HARE, Administrative Assistant
MARIE KIRKEGAARD, Program Officer
BENJAMIN RUSEK, Senior Program Officer

Reviewers

This Consensus Study Report was reviewed in draft form by individuals chosen for their diverse perspectives and technical expertise. The purpose of this independent review is to provide candid and critical comments that will assist the National Academies of Sciences, Engineering, and Medicine in making each consensus study as sound as possible and to ensure that it meets the institutional standards for quality, objectivity, evidence, and responsiveness to the charge. The review comments and draft manuscript remain confidential to protect the integrity of the process.

We thank the following individuals for their review of this report:

DAVID ALDOUS (NAS), University of California, Berkeley
DAVID S.C. CHU, Institute for Defense Analyses
DEBRA DECKER, Stimson Center
ROBIN L. DILLON-MERRILL, Georgetown University
MARTIN E. HELLMAN (NAE), Stanford University
DAVID M. HIGDON, Virginia Polytechnic Institute and State University
JENNIFER LERNER, Harvard University
HERBERT S. LIN, Stanford University
ROGER McCLELLAN (NAM), Independent Consultant
KATHERINE A. McGRADY, CNA
NANCY JO NICHOLAS, Los Alamos National Laboratory
DETLOF VON WINTERFELDT, University of Southern California

Although the reviewers listed above provided many constructive comments and suggestions, they were not asked to endorse the content of the report nor did they see the final draft before its release. The review of this report was overseen by CHRIS G. WHIPPLE (NAE), ENVIRON (retired), and GEORGE APOSTOLAKIS (NAE), Massachusetts Institute of Technology. They were responsible for making certain that an independent examination of this report was carried out in accordance with the standards of the National Academies and that all review comments were carefully considered. Responsibility for the final content rests entirely with the authoring committee and the National Academies.

Contents

APPENDIXES

Preface

This report was mandated by the National Defense Authorization Act for Fiscal Year 2020, which directed the Department of Defense to contract with the National Academies of Sciences, Engineering, and Medicine (the National Academies) to explore the nature and the use of risk analysis methods in assessing nuclear war and nuclear terrorism risks.

The congressional mandate required the National Academies to appoint a committee to address the task in two phases. Phase I of the study is to develop an unclassified report based on access to unclassified information, focusing primarily on a study of risk analysis methods that might be used in assessing the risks of nuclear war and nuclear terrorism. Phase II will expand the focus to include an analysis of the role that the methods and assumptions in risk analysis may play in U.S. security strategy, and it is expected to produce a classified report along with an unclassified summary. The current report is the result of Phase I.

Some readers may ask why this Phase I report does not cover an in-depth analysis of the risks of nuclear war given the Russian Federation invasion of Ukraine. The statement of task for this report is clear in its call for a study of risk analysis methods that might be used in assessing the risks of nuclear war or nuclear terrorism. It is not the charter of this committee to actually conduct its own risk analysis, whether of the risks of nuclear weapons employment in the conflict in Ukraine or in other scenarios associated with nuclear war or nuclear terrorism. The actual risk analysis is in the domain of risk analysis professionals and policy makers in the

Executive Branch. It is possible, however, that the Phase II classified portion of the committee's work may explore further some aspects of different methods of analysis of the nuclear risks associated with the current Ukrainian conflict.

We thank all committee members for their significant contributions to this challenging study. We are most grateful for their candor and collegiality. We would further like to thank the National Academies staff co-directors Carl-Gustav Anderson and Jenny Heimberg. We also thank Michelle Schwalbe for her assistance in the report review process.

Bill Ostendorff and Elisabeth Paté-Cornell, *Co-Chairs*
Committee on Risk Analysis Methods for
Nuclear War and Nuclear Terrorism

Summary

The assessment of risk is complex and often controversial. It is derived from the existence of a hazard, and it is characterized by the uncertainty of possible undesirable events and their outcomes. Few outcomes are as undesirable as nuclear war and nuclear terrorism. Over the decades, much has been written about particular situations, policies, and weapons that might affect the risks of nuclear war and nuclear terrorism. The nature of the concerns and the risk analysis methods used to evaluate them have evolved considerably over time.

In recognition of the risks that both nuclear war and nuclear terrorism pose, the National Defense Authorization Act for Fiscal Year 2020 directed the Department of Defense to contract with the National Academies of Sciences, Engineering, and Medicine to undertake a study to explore the nature of risk analysis methods and their use in assessing nuclear war and nuclear terrorism risks.

This report represents the first phase of the study, which discusses risks, explores the risk assessment literature, highlights the strengths and weaknesses of risk assessment approaches,[1] and discusses some publicly available assumptions that underpin U.S. security strategies, all in the context of nuclear war and nuclear terrorism. The second phase of the study will expand the focus to include an analysis of the role that the assumptions and methods in risk analysis may play in U.S. security strategy. Phase II of the study will produce a classified report and an unclassified summary. Table S-1 details the committee's work.

[1] The terms "risk assessment" and "risk analysis" are used interchangeably in this report.

TABLE S-1 The Phase I and Phase II Committee Tasks

Phase I	Task 1	Identify risks associated with nuclear terrorism and nuclear war.
	Task 2	Explore the prior literature relevant to assessing risks of nuclear terrorism and nuclear war.
	Task 3	Assess the role that quantitative and nonquantitative analytical methods can play in estimating such risks, including the limitations of such analysis.
	Task 4	Identify and examine the assumptions about nuclear risks that underlie the national security strategy of the United States. Task 4 is only partly addressed in Phase I, which considered only assumptions stated in official unclassified documents. Some other assumptions are classified and will be examined in Phase II of the study.
Phase II[a]	Task 5	Describe the consequences or impacts of the methods and assumptions that have been, are, or could be used in developing the nuclear security strategy of the United States.

[a] Phase II may revisit Tasks 1–4, as needed, to address Task 5.

It is important to note that the study does not include performing a risk analysis in either phase of its work. This report will also not address current geopolitical events, such as Russia's 2022 invasion of Ukraine, although these events illustrate the importance of understanding nuclear risks during international conflicts.

The U.S. government and international community have invested significant resources and time in trying to understand and reduce the risks of nuclear war and nuclear terrorism. The current commander of U.S. Strategic Command, as well as campaigners for nuclear disarmament, have asserted that the risks of nuclear war remain very real. Similar statements have been made about the risks of nuclear and radiological terrorism. Moreover, the risks are becoming more complex as new technologies and new adversaries arise.

To identify the threats and consequences associated with nuclear terrorism and nuclear war, an analyst would confront numerous challenges while conducting a risk analysis of nuclear war or nuclear terrorism. The committee identified seven classes of scenarios that might lead to nuclear war: preventive, preemptive, escalatory, catalytic, accidental, unauthorized, and misinformed. The committee also identified three classes of scenarios that might lead to nuclear terrorism: improvised nuclear device, radiological dispersal device or radiological exposure device, and sabotage of a nuclear facility. These classes of scenarios are not mutually exclusive as other interactions among categories could also occur, such as between accidental and misinformed scenarios. These dependencies have to be reflected in any assessment of the risks. The classes of scenarios identified by the committee are used here as examples and are not collectively exhaustive; however, an analyst will have to include all classes of scenarios that they can envision so that the risk results are not underestimated. Estimates of the immediate physical consequences from the use of nuclear weapons have relied on mathematical models based on nuclear physics, past experience, nuclear test data, and other available information. Much is known about some of the physical effects of nuclear weapons (such as immediate estimates of injuries and deaths), though some effects (such as fires, damage in modern urban environments, electromagnetic pulse effects, and climatic effects such as nuclear winter) are not yet well known or difficult to quantify (Frankel et al. 2015). Methods for assessing societal, psychological, and longer-term effects of the use of nuclear weapons have relied heavily on surrogate data for human behavior in response to other catastrophic events.[2] Analyses that use these methods typically contain large uncertainties and strong interdependencies.

The committee examined the history of risk assessments and analyses related to nuclear war and nuclear terrorism, including an exploration of historical attempts to understand the risks of nuclear war and nuclear terrorism, as well as the significant sources of uncertainties involved in assessing the overall risks of nuclear war and nuclear terrorism. Key insights from the historical literature are reflected throughout this report, but a notable gap is the lack of knowledge about the less-well-understood physical effects of nuclear weapons, as well as the assessment and estimation of psychological, societal, and political consequences of nuclear weapons use.

Risk information can be a crucial input for decision makers when making a variety of decisions, including the identification of priorities, the development of new policies or procedures, and the allocation of resources or time. In both natural and engineered systems, especially when statistical data are available and reliable, risk analysis based on frequencies in samples of events can readily produce estimates of future risks. As noted in previous National Academies studies, however, the application of traditional risk methodologies for nuclear war and nuclear terrorism—with limited direct evidence; great uncertainties in contexts; and intelligent, adaptive adversaries (NASEM 2016; National Research Council 2008, 2011)—represents a significant challenge. Among many assumptions, assessments of risks in such contexts have to account for the intentions and interests of the actors, their capabilities, the information and intelligence available to them, and their adaptive responses—all of which may be difficult to assess.

[2] Surrogate data are information about similar phenomena but often from a different context.

The committee considered risk to refer to four key questions[3]:

1. What can happen? Specifically, what can go wrong?
2. How likely is it that these events will happen?
3. If these events happen, what are the potential consequences?
4. What is the time horizon in which these events might happen?

Risk analysis can be a powerful tool for clarifying assumptions; structuring and systematizing thinking about complex, interrelated factors; describing uncertainties; and identifying what further evidence or information might be needed to inform the decisions to be made. However, using risk analysis methods to assess the overall risks of nuclear war and nuclear terrorism is difficult for several reasons.

In addition to the specific conclusions detailed in the body of this report (and listed in Chapter 8), the committee reached three overall conclusions.

1. *Past examples of nuclear war and nuclear terrorism are rare. As such, there is little direct evidence that can be relied on to make empirical estimates about the probability of either.*

Analysts attempt to describe the resulting uncertainties by applying different methods and using multiple sources of information to supplement this limited body of evidence. Similarly, the historical record includes limited examples of attempts at nuclear or radiological terrorism, and analyses of the risks of nuclear terrorism often draw on these. The uncertainties introduced by limited direct evidence are compounded by the important role that human intentions, perceptions, and motivations play. The policy relevance of an overall risk analysis is unclear, given the significant uncertainties involved and the different possible risk attitudes of the decision makers.

While much is known about the physical consequences of nuclear and radiological weapons, the indirect consequences are not as well understood. This includes the social, economic, political, infrastructure, climate, and psychological effects, which are affected by the immediate physical effects of these weapons.

The dynamic interactions among these factors are complex, and methods of analysis for them are less developed. The minimal direct evidence about these effects represents a challenge for assessing the consequences of nuclear weapons used by a state or a terrorist. Even the bombings of Hiroshima and Nagasaki offer only limited information about the likelihood and consequences of conflicts involving modern nuclear weapons.

[3] Questions 1–3 are adapted from Kaplan and Garrick (1981). Question 4 is adapted from Paté-Cornell (2011).

Information elicited from experts is often all that is available for assessing some of the risks associated with nuclear war and nuclear terrorism. Analysts and decision makers need to be aware of the sources of that information, of the biases and limitations that the experts could introduce in the analysis, and of the resulting effects of this information on the risk results. Best practices for expert elicitation can be adapted from other risk analysis disciplines, although some aspects of nuclear war and nuclear terrorism may pose challenges for the adequate application of these methods.

2. *The scenarios that might lead to nuclear war and nuclear terrorism are numerous and involve many interdependent factors, and the assessment of their risks often depends on the capabilities, values, perceptions, and intentions of many experts and actors.*

The risks of nuclear war and nuclear terrorism depend in part on the effectiveness of deterrence, which reflects the capabilities, beliefs, motivations, intentions, anticipation strategies, and information available to all parties involved. The unavailability and inaccuracy of information in the throes of a crisis can potentially increase the risks faced by both aggressors and defenders. The risks of nuclear war and nuclear terrorism scenarios vary in terms of the justification or initiating reason by states or actors involved, the type and number of weapons used, and the target(s), among many other highly interdependent factors. Because there are a large number of scenario possibilities, they are often grouped together and analyzed as classes of scenarios that share some key common factors.

Assessing the overall risks of nuclear war and nuclear terrorism involves great uncertainties about the likelihood and consequences of different scenarios. The assessment and communications of these uncertainties are critical for policy decisions essential to managing these risks. However, the value of risk analysis is not solely in assessing the overall risks. Risk analysis can provide valuable input on many smaller-scale problems related to nuclear war and nuclear terrorism. Many analyses are intended to determine the relative or comparative risks of classes of scenarios (e.g., the risk of sabotage of a nuclear facility compared with the risk of a radiological exposure device; or the determination of the risk reductions associated with different investments or design changes) or to address specific questions confronting decision makers such as: What is the reliability of a particular country's nuclear stockpile? What is the probability that a particular model of detector at an automobile border crossing will detect a specific level of radiation? Which nuclear facilities should be inspected and how often? For risk management problems that involve significant uncertainties and a need to make resource-constrained decisions, assessing the risk variations associated with different options can help inform decision making.

Analysts inevitably make assumptions in risk analysis, including assumptions about the definition and the framing of the risk problem; which models can be used effectively; the reliability of data; and the capabilities, intent, and potential actions of adversaries. Strategic assumptions can help define the boundaries of a risk problem. Some strategic assumptions address the nature or magnitude of risks, the effect of risk drivers, whether policies or actions increase or decrease the risks, the nature and the variety of threats that confront the United States, and the most likely scenarios. Strategic assumptions also include risks of nuclear wars outside the borders of the United States.

3. *Different risk assessment methods are more or less suited to different situations and goals.*

The committee identified the following methods relevant to analyzing these risks and considered the applicability and limitations of those methods:

- *First-strike stability analyses* compare the advantages to both sides of striking first in a crisis in which nuclear war appears imminent.
- *Probabilistic risk assessment* can explore interactions between adaptive adversaries, though extracting qualitative values from quantitative outputs may obscure some of the nuanced results.
- *Order-of-magnitude estimates* set extreme bounds on the probability of a nuclear incident, which can then be incrementally narrowed.
- *Game theory* can be used to model potential moves and their outcomes between intelligent adversaries based on information about their preferences and capabilities.
- *Adversarial risk analysis* can be used to evaluate possible choices of an intelligent adversary or small number of adversaries.
- *Agent-based models* can estimate behaviors of individuals given defined rules and uncertainties.
- *Multi-attribute models* assess the different elements (attributes) of the outcomes of different scenarios, according to defined and weighted criteria among the different attributes of the decision makers' preferences.
- *Network models* use network analysis to explore multiple alternatives at nodes representing key events and scenarios in the path from start to end.
- *Nuclear and conventional force exchange models* can help assess deterrence by quantifying the outcomes of potential nuclear or conventional attacks.

Just as the structure, parameters, and assumptions in a risk analysis may color the results of a risk analysis, the ways that risk information is assessed, framed, or presented has a powerful effect on how that information is understood and used in decisions. Risk analysis results are most valuable when the methods and assumptions by which they were generated is clear, the process is replicable, trust in the analytical process is established, and the results address the real questions or decisions that the decision makers are facing.

Risk information may be a valuable input to decision making, but it does not and cannot dictate decisions, which also depend on preferences and risk attitudes. Other considerations beyond risk need to be taken into account, such as legal, political, or budgetary consequences and constraints. Emerging technologies, such as new weapons systems and advances with artificial intelligence, are quickly changing the risk and deterrence landscape. The U.S. nuclear posture has evolved over time, taking into account new threats, developing deterrence strategies involving different U.S. adversaries, technological advancements, nuclear arms treaties, and changing geopolitical environments. U.S. assessments of the risks of nuclear terrorism have likewise evolved over time, taking into account new threats and emerging technologies.

As the context in which decisions about nuclear war and nuclear terrorism are made continues to evolve, risk assessment will continue to be a valuable tool for analysts and decision makers.

1

Introduction

This report was mandated by the National Defense Authorization Act for Fiscal Year 2020 (P.L. 116-92), which directed the Department of Defense (DoD) to contract with the National Academies of Sciences, Engineering, and Medicine (the National Academies) to explore the nature and the use of risk analysis methods in assessing nuclear war and nuclear terrorism risks. The National Academies appointed the Committee on Risk Analysis Methods for Nuclear War and Nuclear Terrorism to carry out this work.

COMMITTEE TASK AND SCOPE OF WORK

The formal task for the committee is shown in Box 1-1. The request required the committee to address the work in two phases. Phase I of the study is to develop an unclassified report based on access to unclassified information and primarily focuses on the nature and the use of analytical methods to assess the risks of nuclear terrorism and nuclear war. Phase II expands the focus to include an analysis of the role that the methods and assumptions in risk analysis may play in U.S. security strategy[1]; this phase is expected to produce a classified report along with an unclassified summary. The current report is the product of Phase I.

To carry out the Phase I assessment, the National Academies appointed a committee of 14 members with expertise covering risk analysis, decision analysis,

[1] Phase II may also require the committee to revisit tasks addressed in Phase I, as needed and after the committee has access to classified information.

BOX 1-1
Statement of Task

The National Academies of Sciences, Engineering, and Medicine will convene an ad hoc committee of experts to examine whether a risk assessment framework is applicable to determining the potential risks of nuclear terrorism and nuclear war; and to examine assumptions in nuclear policy and doctrine and their implications on national security. During this examination, the committee will undertake the following:

1. Identify risks associated with nuclear terrorism and nuclear war;
2. Explore the prior literature relevant to assessing risks of nuclear terrorism and nuclear war;
3. Assess the role that quantitative and nonquantitative analytical methods can play in estimating such risks, including the limitations of such analysis;
4. Identify and examine the assumptions about nuclear risks that underlie the national security strategy of the United States; and
5. Describe the consequences or impacts of the methods and assumptions that have been, are, or could be used in developing the nuclear security strategy of the United States.

The committee will issue an unclassified report which may include findings and recommendations regarding the use of analytical methods to assess the risks of nuclear terrorism and nuclear war.

At the conclusion of the study, the committee will issue a final report that expands upon the use of analytical methods to assess the risks of nuclear terrorism and nuclear war and the role such approaches may play in U.S. security strategy. This final report may include findings and recommendations supported by classified information.

system modeling, strategy development, risk perception, social and behavioral science, and the analysis of nuclear war and nuclear terrorism. Committee biographies are provided in Appendix E.[2]

The committee held several data-gathering meetings in support of Phase I: their agendas are shown in Appendix D. At its first meeting, the committee was briefed on the origin of the study and expectations for its use by staff from the Armed Services Committee of the U.S. House of Representatives, the DoD Office of the Under Secretary of Defense for Policy, and the U.S. Strategic Command. In later meetings the committee learned about methods of risk analysis related to nuclear war and nuclear terrorism that have been used previously or are currently used in the U.S. government and academia. The committee also heard from some U.S. government decision makers on how they use the output of risk analysis to inform

[2] A subset of the committee and National Academies staff with appropriate clearances will conduct the classified Phase II part of the study.

their decisions. Details on current U.S. government risk analysis methods and the assumptions made in these analyses were not available for Phase I of the study and limited the committee's review of those methods.

In the unclassified domain of its Phase I study, the committee did not find a clearly defined U.S. government-wide program assessing the risks of nuclear terrorism or nuclear war. Therefore, as the consequences of nuclear catastrophe affect virtually all aspects of society and government, from medical care, food supply, energy, and communications to economic, psychological, and political responses, the committee instead provides examples of various risk analysis techniques that could support different risk management efforts. In principle, these methods could be applied to analyzing the risks of nuclear war and nuclear terrorism. One of the committee's objectives was to highlight the applicability and limitations of relevant risk analysis methods.

It is essential to note that the statement of task does not require the committee to perform a risk analysis,[3] but to focus on the *methods* of risk analysis. To describe these methods, the committee presents examples in this report—for instance, of risk scenarios—but these should not be considered an exhaustive description of the possibilities.

It is also important to note that the statement of task focuses on risk analysis. Risk analysis and risk assessment are often used interchangeably, as they are in this report.

AUDIENCE FOR THIS REPORT

This report was written with the intention of informing Congress, DoD, decision makers, policy makers, risk analysts in U.S. government departments and agencies, and the interested public on how risk analysis is or could be performed and how complex problems—such as the risks of nuclear war or nuclear terrorism—might be better understood through careful analysis. It is also intended to highlight the limitations of these approaches. In addition, the committee hopes to inform those conducting nuclear risk analyses on challenges and best practices to follow and on potential improvements of these practices.

COMMITTEE INTERPRETATION OF THE STATEMENT OF TASK

The committee viewed its overarching task as determining whether analytical methods or techniques are applicable to assessing the potential risks of nuclear terrorism and nuclear war. In Phase I, the committee focused on Tasks 1 through

[3] This is especially important to note as this report was being written during the war between Russia and Ukraine, which led to questions about the use of nuclear weapons.

4 in Box 1-1, described here in detail along with the committee's approach to addressing each. Phase II will provide an opportunity for further analysis of Tasks 1 through 4, as well as the committee's examination of Task 5, supported by classified information. This report will not address current geopolitical events, such as Russia's 2022 invasion of Ukraine, although these events illustrate the importance of understanding nuclear risks before and during international conflicts.

Task 1 calls for the committee to identify risks associated with nuclear terrorism and nuclear war in both the United States and the rest of the world. The committee did not attempt to develop an exhaustive list of risks associated with nuclear war or terrorism. Rather, in Chapter 2, the committee describes the current geopolitical context, some illustrative classes of scenarios, and what is known about the consequences of the use of nuclear weapons.

The committee decided to treat "nuclear war" and "nuclear terrorism" as two separate topics, although the committee recognized that some scenarios and cases involve both nuclear war and nuclear terrorism and that there is an overlap in analytical methods to examine issues in both terrorism and war. When appropriate, the committee has identified techniques that are relevant to questions and decisions related to both nuclear terrorism and nuclear war. Chapter 2 separately lists classes of scenarios for nuclear terrorism and for nuclear war, as an example of the types of risks that could be explored. These examples are intended as one organizing principle that might be applied, but a comprehensive analysis of relevant scenarios is the task of risk analysts. As noted above, the committee's statement of task did not call for an attempt to estimate the risks of nuclear war or the risks of nuclear terrorism but, rather, the methods that can be used to do so. The committee offers these general classes of scenarios as one possible approach to analyzing the risks related to nuclear war and nuclear terrorism; some questions and decisions will be amenable to other organizing principles.

Task 2 asks the committee to explore prior literature relevant to assessing the risks of nuclear terrorism and nuclear war. Key insights from this literature are presented in Chapter 3.

Task 3 calls for the committee to assess the role that quantitative and non-quantitative analytical methods can play in estimating the risks of nuclear war and nuclear terrorism, including the potential insights and limitations of risk analysis techniques. This task is central to Phase I of the report. To address this task, Chapter 4 describes the major challenges and sources of uncertainty relevant to assessing the overall risks of nuclear war and nuclear terrorism. This chapter also describes what is currently known about the consequences of nuclear weapons use related to the scenarios described, ranging from the detonation of a single small weapon to large-scale nuclear war.

In Chapter 5, the committee addresses the use of risk analysis methods to support specific decisions related to the management of the risks of nuclear war and nuclear terrorism. Chapter 6 details the applicability and limitations of methods of risk analysis. Chapter 7 discusses the role of decision makers in risk and decision analyses, as well as the importance of communication of risk analysis results. Chapter 8 provides a summary of the key conclusions throughout the report. Several appendixes offer additional information.

Task 4 directs the committee to identify and examine the assumptions about nuclear risks that underlie the national security strategy of the United States. To address this task, the committee identified text within publicly available U.S. documents related to nuclear security strategy that included stated assumptions about risks: a sample of them are shown in Appendix A. This list is neither complete nor definitive, and it may not fully reflect U.S. government capabilities and positions. The representative set of nuclear risk assumptions underlying U.S. government strategy will be revisited during Phase II of the committee's work. Appendix B offers a short discussion of uncertainties both aleatory (randomness) and epistemic (systematic, due to limited knowledge). Appendix C summarizes U.S. government policy-making structure as it relates to nuclear war and nuclear terrorism.

2

The Threat of Nuclear War and Nuclear Terrorism: Classes of Scenarios

Scenarios play a critical role in scoping a risk analysis. A scenario, such as those described in this chapter, is the conjunction of events and system states that describes a situation and its possible paths of evolution so that one can then evaluate the potential risks associated with it. This chapter identifies some classes of scenarios of nuclear war and nuclear terrorism for illustrative purposes.

In developing scenarios, analysts are confronted with a fundamental question: How complex should the scenario description be? Scenarios can be made extremely complex by adding details that may not be fully relevant, to the point at which their likelihood becomes very small with the addition of each detail or component. Scenario specificity is a balancing act: analysts have to balance identifying groups of scenarios in a description that is simple enough that it can be analyzed and, at the same time, includes all the essential components that will make the results relevant.

Forecasting geopolitics is obviously difficult (Scoblic and Tetlock 2020), and the following classes of scenarios are not intended as an exhaustive set. Many other scenarios are possible, and multiple scenarios could unfold simultaneously. Rather, the committee offers these general classes of scenarios as one possible approach to organizing risk analyses related to nuclear war and nuclear terrorism.

DEVICE TYPES AND SCALES OF EVENTS

Devices used in nuclear war and nuclear terrorism can be grouped into those in which a nuclear detonation occurs and those in which it does not. Devices in which a nuclear detonation occurs can occur in both nuclear terrorism and war scenarios. These nuclear weapons range from a terrorist-constructed improvised nuclear device or a terrorist-produced or -obtained nuclear weapon (stolen or clandestinely provided by a state) to state-developed tactical or strategic nuclear weapons. The scale of these weapons can be listed notionally from lowest to highest yield, from a fraction of a kiloton to tens of megatons.

Devices or events in which a nuclear detonation does not occur are typically related to nuclear or radiological terrorism scenarios; they include radiological dispersal devices, radiological exposure devices, and nuclear facility sabotage. The scales of destruction of these events are thought to be localized (e.g., to a city or a region) but they could have large economic, social, and psychological consequences. "Success" for a terrorist could be to create fear and may not include the release of any radioactivity.

CLASSES OF NUCLEAR WAR SCENARIOS

The risks of a conflict that involves nuclear weapons is driven by the capabilities and intentions of adversaries. Sources of tension between states with nuclear weapons, the potential for escalation from conventional warfare, cross-domain instability (e.g., crisis in space or cyber domains leading to a nuclear response), and alliance commitments can each play a role in triggering nuclear war. Many other factors are also important, such as alert status and force structure.

There are many imaginable scenarios that would involve the use of nuclear weapons between states. To help identify the risks associated with nuclear war, the following set of classes of nuclear war scenarios is presented as a possible approach to organizing classes of scenarios. If analysts intend to determine the overall risks of nuclear war, they will need to address the completeness of the set of scenario classes, the completeness of scenarios within classes, and their interdependencies and underlying assumptions.

As noted above, the classes of nuclear wars identified by the committee are not exhaustive; moreover, individual scenarios may have attributes of more than one class.

Preventive Nuclear War

The idea that a preventive nuclear war against a nonnuclear or a nascent nuclear state would prevent it from starting a nuclear war in the future has been considered, but has never been carried out. Yet future scenarios of that kind could lead to actual nuclear use.

Preemptive Nuclear War

Preemptive nuclear war refers to an instance in which an actor strikes first due to the fear that, if it does not do so, the other side will strike first or it believes it can achieve a significant advantage by striking first. Concerns about preemption were the focus of first-strike stability analyses throughout much of the Cold War.

Escalatory Nuclear War

Escalatory nuclear war refers to an instance in which ongoing conventional military conflict leads one side to initiate the use of nuclear weapons. This escalation can be either strategic, to achieve a broader goal, or tactical, to accomplish a specific mission. The threat of escalation to nuclear war is both a crisis management tool and a risk. The incentives to escalate to higher levels of violence in a conflict can arise from particular geographies, the vulnerability of military forces and command and control to enemy attack, fear of losing a conflict, evolving technologies that may create advantages (e.g., cyber and counter-space weaponry), and technologies and circumstances that reduce the time for decisions.

Catalytic Nuclear War

Catalytic nuclear war generally refers to an instance when a state initiates the use of nuclear weapons because it or one of its allies to whom it has made a firm deterrent commitment faces an existential threat from nonnuclear weapons. If the number of nuclear states increases and as nonnuclear states continue to rely on an ally's nuclear umbrella, the possibility of catalytic nuclear war could potentially increase.

Accidental Nuclear War

Accidental nuclear war refers to instances when an unintended mishap inadvertently leads to war. Unforeseeable accidents are considered inherent characteristics of complex systems (Perrow 2011). Some complex systems and processes can be safer than simple ones if they involve effective checking processes and properly designed redundancies.

Unauthorized Nuclear War

Unauthorized nuclear war refers to an instance when the decision to use nuclear weapons is made by a subordinate without his or her leadership's direction.

The delegation of launch authority may enhance deterrence, but it simultaneously increases the risks of an unauthorized nuclear war.

Misinformed Nuclear War

Misinformed nuclear war refers to an instance when leaders act on erroneous information or faulty analysis. A launch of nuclear-armed missiles, based on a false warning of an attack, would be an example of this category.

CLASSES OF NUCLEAR TERRORISM SCENARIOS

As with nuclear war, the many scenarios involving the use of radiological or nuclear weapons by terrorists can be classified into categories and analyzed to set priorities to deter, detect, and respond to nuclear threats. Below are three broad classes of scenarios: those involving stolen or otherwise acquired weapons or improvised nuclear devices, those involving radiological dispersal devices or radiological exposure devices, and those involving the sabotage of major nuclear facilities. Here again, the committee offers this organization of classes of scenarios to assist in identifying the risks of nuclear terrorism, but it is important to note that some questions and decisions may be better informed by organizing the classes of scenarios differently.

Acquired Weapons or Improvised Nuclear Devices

Scenarios in this class would require terrorists to gain access to special nuclear materials (plutonium and highly enriched uranium) with which to build a device or to gain access to a nuclear weapon either by stealing one or by complicity. Scenarios in this class might also include details related to the transportation and successful use of improvised nuclear devices.

Radiological Dispersal Devices and Radiological Exposure Devices

With radiological dispersal devices, radioactivity is distributed through the environment either using explosives ("dirty bombs") or other methods. With radiological exposure devices, the radioactive source remains contained (rather than dispersed in the environment). Exposure can be significant, but would only occur when people are near the source.

Sabotage of Major Nuclear Facilities

The sabotage of a nuclear installations could lead to widespread contamination, access to nuclear material, and a general sense of panic, which was seen in the Russian seizure of Ukraine's Chernobyl and Zaporizhzhia nuclear facilities. Sabotage can happen by intrusion or by complicity of an insider. In general, an attack on a nuclear facility cannot result in a nuclear explosion but rather in radioactive dispersal (World Nuclear Association 2021). The nuclear fissile material, if dispersed, poses direct radiological hazard due to exposure, and it can lead to contamination of the environment, including soil, atmosphere, built structures, and vegetation that can then be ingested. It can also lead to human exposure. High exposure levels can cause both short-term illness and death, as well as longer-term deaths from cancer and other diseases. The Chernobyl disaster provides an illustration of the extent of contamination and its long-term effects—some less expected, such as the reemergence of nature and the life of the few people who refused to evacuate. A nuclear power plant typically contains tons of radioactive material, in comparison with a nuclear weapon that contains on the order of tens of kilograms, and disruption of a gigawatt power plant can produce radioactive contamination of a severity comparable to that of a megaton explosion (Eisenbud and Gesell 1997).

In a National Research Council (2006) study, five possible attack scenarios were identified: (1) ground attack by a group of well-trained individuals, (2) air attack using a civilian aircraft or a smaller private aircraft carrying explosives, (3) attacks involving combined air and land attacks, (4) attack by a combination of sea and land, and (5) theft of spent fuel by terrorists to produce a dispersal device. In addition to attacks on the facility structures that contain the reactor, deliberate actions that lead to a fire in a spent fuel pool could be especially devastating due to widespread dispersal of radioactive material through a smoke plume (National Research Council 2006). The general view is that aircraft-based attacks on U.S. nuclear facilities will not cause dispersal due to the installed containment structures and missile shields.

In addition to sabotage events that could release radioactive materials, terrorists' objectives may be focused on social or psychological effects—creating fear or panic or damaging public trust in or the reputation of the entity managing the nuclear facility—without the intention of releasing any radioactive materials (e.g., Y-12 protester break-in in 2012 [GAO 2014]).

3

The History and Literature of Risk Assessment for Nuclear War and Nuclear Terrorism

This chapter reviews the key research in the assessment of the risks of nuclear war and nuclear terrorism. It provides an overview of major developments and insights, with a primary focus on U.S. policy and risk assessment.

THE HISTORY AND LITERATURE OF RISK ASSESSMENT FOR NUCLEAR WAR

Over the decades, much has been written about the risks of nuclear war or how particular situations, policies, or weapons might affect it. The nature of the concerns and the methods used to evaluate them have evolved over the decades.

1940s and 1950s

In the years immediately following World War II, there was widespread concern that future wars could lead to unprecedented devastation. The U.S. military was still determining how best to use nuclear weapons and developing internal capabilities to make those assessments. The United States quickly moved from a position of nuclear "unipolarity" (holding a monopoly on nuclear weapons and delivery systems) to a bipolar position as the Soviet Union developed nuclear weapons and the means to deliver them.

Early on, some analysts envisioned that nuclear weapons would create such fear that they might prevent future wars. While the concept of deterrence has long been relevant to conventional conflict, the presence of nuclear weapons changed the deterrence landscape (Brodie 1946).

The RAND Corporation (established in 1948) led the development of much of the early U.S. thinking about nuclear strategy and ways to assess different elements of nuclear risks, including a proposal to effectively study the risk of nuclear war to help guide U.S. weapons choices in the context of various war types. The analysis was guided by identification of different scenarios and methods (Ansoff et al. 1951; Wohlstetter 1952; Wohlstetter and Rowen 1952).

RAND's analysis of nuclear weapons capabilities and vulnerabilities to Soviet surprise attack began early in the Cold War (Freedman 2003). By 1956, the analysts had assessed the vulnerability of U.S. facilities to a Soviet intercontinental ballistic missile attack. This analysis was used in introducing the concepts of *first* and *second strikes* into strategic theory (Freedman 2003; RAND 1956). A first strike would begin a nuclear war with the intent of crippling the enemy's nuclear capabilities and hence its means of retaliation. A second strike would be the retaliation after absorbing an enemy first strike.

Detailed methods were developed to assess the vulnerability of particular weapon deployments to various types of attack and to assess the effectiveness of potential U.S. attacks on Soviet targets. These technical strategic exchange calculations came to underpin much U.S. thinking about nuclear war. While Soviet analysts also performed calculations about the vulnerability of forces and the effectiveness of potential strikes, overall Soviet assessments tended to be more focused on broader geopolitical issues, what the Soviets referred to as the global "correlation of forces" (Sokolovskii et al. 1963).

After a great deal of work on the survivability of U.S. forces, Schelling (1958) raised the concern that the vulnerability of Soviet forces to U.S. attacks could, paradoxically, undermine U.S. security as well. If both sides thought they would be better off if they struck first and destroyed a large portion of the other side's nuclear forces, and if both sides feared that the other side was thinking the same, Schelling hypothesized that this would increase the risk that one country would decide to attack in a crisis. Schelling's paper established the concept that came to be known as first-strike stability: if both sides had survivable forces, neither side would have an incentive to strike first, and the nuclear balance would be more stable. While U.S. arms control advocates adopted this idea, arguing that both sides' security would benefit if both avoided seriously threatening the other's nuclear forces, in reality, the militaries on both sides continued to pursue the ability to attack each other's nuclear forces and continue to do so today.

In this era, game theory was used to think through circumstances in which one side or the other might have an incentive to carry out a nuclear strike or agree to and comply with a particular agreement (Dresher 1951; Haywood 1954; Schelling 1980).

The 1960s

Two events in the early 1960s focused attention on the real possibility of nuclear war: the Berlin Crisis of 1961 (DOS 1966) and the Cuban missile crisis in 1962 (Allison and Zelikow 1999). These events transformed concepts of nuclear war into very realistic possibilities to the public and affected the U.S. government's thinking about nuclear threats. During this period, the Kennedy administration introduced the concept of a limited response that would reduce the quantity of weapons launched in response to an initial attack (Ellsberg 2017).

During the 1960s, exchange calculations of the sort initiated in the 1950s became more sophisticated and addressed new issues, producing estimates of the probability of destroying hardened targets (such as missile silos) with weapons of varying accuracy, and the probability of penetrating missile defenses. (Hardened sites began to be tested and deployed by the late 1960s.)

The late 1950s and early 1960s marked the beginning of the U.S. "triad" of nuclear delivery vehicles with different operational advantages:

- Intercontinental ballistic missiles had accuracy and prompt responsiveness to attack Soviet hardened targets (e.g., weapon silos).
- Submarine-launched ballistic missiles were considered survivable because of the difficulty in identifying their location while submerged on nuclear deterrent patrol and thus able to retaliate.
- Land-based bombers could be dispersed quickly to different bases and recalled if the crisis deescalated; they could be launched on warning and return to base under "fail safe" procedures if the warning turned out to be a false alarm.

The United States also deployed thousands of shorter-range nuclear weapons on land and on Navy ships (Woolf 2008).

The Soviet Union adopted a similar approach, which added credibility to the concept of stability arising from mutual assured destruction (Freedman 2003). As nuclear arsenals expanded in the United States and the Soviet Union, stability assessments began to focus not only on crisis stability, but also on arms race stability, including whether the structure of forces was such that either side thought it could get an advantage by expanding its nuclear forces. This thinking led to consideration of how many nuclear weapons the United States should have in its arsenal. Then-Secretary of Defense McNamara announced the idea of assured destruction, whereby the United States needed enough weapons that could survive and retaliate.

Data from nuclear-explosion tests in the 1950s and the 1960s contributed to further analyses of the consequences of nuclear war in the 1960s. Studies of consequences included some of the first analyses of the psychological impact of nuclear weapons (Lifton 1967). Because of the difficulty of assessing the risks of escalating crises or the chance of one side or the other backing down, analysts began to rely more heavily on war games, in which participants would play through various hypothetical crises, trying to understand what circumstances increased or decreased the odds that one side or another would use nuclear weapons.

Game theory continued to be used to understand how countries might respond to nuclear threats. Following the work of Schelling (1960), Kobe (1962) proposed an "autocatalytic" model that provided game theoretical conditions under which one nation would mount a nuclear attack against another, and attendant calculations that estimated the number of consequent deaths.[1] Mathematical theorems on fundamental instability of nuclear multipolarity were also advanced (Aumann et al. 1995; Selten and Tietz 1966).

During the 1960s, concerns over the possibility of unauthorized or accidental use of nuclear weapons began to emerge. Assessments of the danger of unauthorized use relied initially on expert judgment and, later, on systems engineering analysis of the difficulty of overcoming the measures put in place to block such use.

By the late 1960s, a series of accidents involving nuclear weapons (particularly, accidents in which thermonuclear weapons were dropped from aircraft or aircraft crashed carrying such weapons) led to a decision to end the U.S. practice of keeping a small number of bombers armed with nuclear weapons in the air at all times. At the same time, there were substantial improvements in the safety design of U.S. nuclear weapons, including such innovations as primary fission components resistant to fire; "insensitive high explosives" that were much more difficult to detonate accidentally; improved arming and fuzing mechanisms that provided high confidence no detonation signal would be sent accidentally (including systems that blocked arming of the weapon until it had been through the expected flight sequence); and, perhaps most important, "one-point safety," a requirement that the probability of achieving a nuclear yield greater than the equivalent of 4 pounds of TNT in the event of a one-point initiation of the main charge high explosive must not exceed one in a million (DOE 2015). A variety of systems engineering methods based on probabilistic risk assessment were used to assess these safety systems, as similar methods were used in other engineering fields. Few assessments, however, explored in detail how such accidents might lead to nuclear war if they were to occur in a moment of intense crisis (Sagan 1993).

[1] The model required that the number of nuclear powers be greater than or equal to three and that the attacking nation can do so in such a way that the blame for the attack could be shifted to a different nuclear power. Technically, this methodology falls within the scope of this study's charge, but the committee believes the approach is largely irrelevant because of its strong assumptions, its assumption that the attacker could lay the blame at someone else's door (which is challenging given intelligence capabilities), and its lack of a probability statement about nuclear war. (Instead, it identifies a set of nonstochastic conditions under which a game theorist would choose to make a sneak attack.)

The 1960s also saw increasing concern about the spread of nuclear weapons among countries and the possibility that this spread would lead to more danger of nuclear war—including the possibility that other nuclear-armed states might somehow provoke a U.S.-Soviet nuclear war. This concern was heightened by the Chinese nuclear-explosion test in 1964. Ultimately, this concern led to negotiation of the Nuclear Nonproliferation Treaty, which opened for signature in 1968 and has served as the foundation of the global effort to stem the spread of nuclear weapons ever since. Assessments of this "Nth-country problem" relied primarily on expert judgments; wargaming was also used to explore how additional nuclear-armed countries might affect some types of crises.

The 1970s

The 1970s saw important progress in formalizing probabilistic risk assessment techniques, initially for analyses of the safety of nuclear reactors (NRC 1975). Similar analyses of potential pathways to an undesired outcome, with assessments of each step on the pathway, began to be applied in many other engineered systems, including a reliability model for the command and control of U.S. nuclear forces (Paté-Cornell and Neu 1985).

The Strategic Arms Limitation Talks I agreements, the Anti-Ballistic Missile Treaty, and the Interim Agreement on offensive forces were all signed in 1972. The Anti-Ballistic Missile Treaty was intended to improve both arms race and crisis stability. The Interim Agreement's limits—and those of subsequent arms control agreements—offered a degree of predictability and transparency, ultimately reducing hostility between the United States and the Soviet Union. Many assessments explored the pros and cons of different potential arms control provisions, incorporating strategic exchange calculations, intelligence assessments of potential future adversary forces with and without agreed restraints, assessments of verification effectiveness, and the like. Still, critics argued that arms control advocates were seeking agreements for their own sake, more than agreements carefully tailored to increase U.S. security.

In addition to arms control, the United States and the Soviet Union undertook a range of confidence-building measures intended to reduce the risks of armed conflict between them that might escalate to nuclear war.[2] At the end of the decade, President Carter issued Presidential Directive 59, calling for a nuclear strategy that included flexible options, including a heavy emphasis on counterforce attacks on

[2] These measures had begun in the 1960s, after the Cuban missile crisis, with the agreement on establishing a hotline for rapid communication between the United States and the Soviet Union. The measures eventually led to the Prevention of Dangerous Military Activities agreement in the 1980s (Campbell 1991).

Soviet nuclear forces. The United States continued to build up its strategic nuclear forces, with the MX missile, the Trident submarine-launched missile, air-launched cruise missiles, and the B-1 bomber.

The 1970s also saw controversies over extended deterrence and its credibility. The United States' withdrawal from Vietnam and its aftermath led a number of allies to question the reliability of U.S. guarantees. In Europe, there were serious debates over whether the Soviet bloc really had a major conventional advantage over North Atlantic Treaty Organization (NATO) forces, necessitating continued reliance on large numbers of tactical nuclear weapons and plans for early use of them should war break out. Moreover, the Soviet Union began replacing older medium-range missiles with the much more capable three-warhead SS-20 missiles, which were seen by some as posing a new threat to Europe for which the United States had no obvious counter. After considerable debate, in 1979 NATO undertook the "dual-track" decision, under which the United States would deploy Pershing II ballistic missiles and ground-launched cruise missiles in response to the SS-20s, while simultaneously seeking to negotiate an agreement limiting such weapons. A variety of military assessment approaches were used to assess the capabilities of conventional forces on each side and of the nuclear missiles being deployed. However, assessments of how much these deployments might affect the risks of nuclear war are not known to this committee.

The 1970s also saw continuing concern over the potential spread of nuclear weapons and the effect it might have on the overall risks of nuclear war, particularly following India's nuclear test in 1974. The United States began to focus on detecting and stopping nuclear weapons programs in other countries, while both the United States and the Soviet Union worked to convince their allies and nonaligned states to sign the Nuclear Nonproliferation Treaty. China's nuclear forces grew, though they remained quite small, and relatively little U.S. analysis was focused on assessing possibilities of nuclear war with China.

The 1980s

The 1980s saw some of the most intense hostility of the Cold War in the early part of the decade, a shift toward major arms control progress in the middle of the decade, and the beginning of the end of the Soviet Union and its alliance system toward the end of the decade. Assessments of the risks of nuclear war and how best to address them had a difficult time keeping up with the pace of change.

President Reagan came to power supporting a major buildup of U.S. military capabilities to achieve "peace through strength," and he accelerated the increase in investment in U.S. nuclear forces begun in the Carter administration. Strategic exchange calculations and expert judgments were the main methods used to assess what weapons were needed and in what quantities.

The 1980s also saw further elaboration of more limited options in U.S. nuclear war planning. A variety of techniques, including expert judgment, exchange calculations, and wargaming, was used to help inform these plans. Additional attention was paid to improving the survivability of systems for nuclear command and control and for ensuring the continuity of government in the event of nuclear war. New investments were made in a variety of systems for communicating with nuclear forces.

The early 1980s saw an increase in superpower tensions that raised both government and public concerns over the risks of nuclear war. In 1983, the Soviet Union accidentally shot down a civilian airliner (mistaking it for an intelligence aircraft). The same year, Reagan launched the Strategic Defense Initiative, calling on scientists and engineers to develop technology that would render offensive nuclear missiles "impotent and obsolete." Strategic exchange estimates, analyses of potential countermeasures to defenses, and a technical review of the program by the American Physical Society quickly made clear that determining whether the objective of the Strategic Defense Initiative was achievable was at least a decade or more away. But, the program proceeded, with officials sometimes articulating more limited objectives (Bloembergen et al. 1987).

In 1985, Mikhail Gorbachev (who had recently become the general secretary of the Communist Party of the Soviet Union) met with Reagan at a summit in Geneva. The two leaders agreed that neither side would win from a nuclear war and agreed to resume arms control negotiations.

In 1987, Reagan and Gorbachev signed the Intermediate-Range Nuclear Forces Treaty, eliminating the entire class of ground-based missiles (with ranges from 500 to 5,500 kilometers) from their arsenals, including the Soviet SS-20s and a variety of shorter-range systems and the U.S. Pershing II and ground-launched cruise missiles, and incorporating on-site inspections for the first time. The Strategic Arms Reduction Treaty (START), which first called for real reductions in strategic forces on each side, came a few years later.

By this time, assessments of such accords were more complex than they had previously been. A variety of methods—including strategic exchange calculations and engineering and intelligence estimates about the capabilities of particular weapons and how rapidly more of them could be built—were used to assess the degree to which the agreements contributed to crisis stability, improved predictability and strategic force planning, and enhanced transparency of each side's strategic posture. These assessments included analyses of a potential breakout from these agreements and how readily the United States would be able to detect large-scale violations and respond to them to protect its interests.

The 1980s also saw the first analyses that indicated that nuclear war could cause a "nuclear winter" that could interfere with global food production. Gorbachev noted, in particular, that these assessments informed his work toward nuclear arms reductions. The consequences of large-scale nuclear war continued to influence popular culture, with books such as Jonathan Schell's *The Fate of the Earth* (focusing exclusively on the danger of nuclear war) and movies such as *The Day After* (which Reagan noted in his journal left him greatly depressed).

By the end of the 1980s, superpower tensions were significantly reduced, and communist governments were ending in Eastern Europe without the Soviet government intervention. The most dramatic change was the fall of the Berlin wall in 1989.

The 1990s

The risks of nuclear war and U.S. policies to address it were transformed by the collapse of the Soviet Union in 1991. As the Soviet Union neared collapse, President George H.W. Bush concluded that a change in U.S. nuclear policy was needed, and he made far-reaching changes: unilaterally pledging to eliminate all battlefield nuclear weapons, eliminating all nuclear weapons from Navy surface ships and aircraft (leaving only submarine-launched ballistic missiles and sea-launched cruise missiles on submarines), pulling tactical nuclear weapons back to U.S. soil (leaving only air-delivered bombs in Europe), taking U.S. nuclear bombers off strip alert, and de-alerting missiles scheduled for elimination under START. Gorbachev soon followed with unilateral initiatives and, once the Soviet Union ceased to exist and Boris Yeltsin took power as president of the Russian Federation, he reconfirmed Gorbachev's initiatives and added others.

One early U.S. response to the Soviet collapse was the Cooperative Threat Reduction program and related efforts in the U.S. Department of State, in which the United States provided funding to work cooperatively with Russia and the other states of the former Soviet Union (and, eventually, elsewhere) to dismantle and secure the nuclear, biological, and chemical weapons and materials remaining from the Cold War.[3] Few, if any, unclassified assessments sought to understand how these initiatives affected the risks of nuclear war; rather, attention was focused on engineering, cost, and political assessments of particular projects and how they could best be accomplished.

In 1992, the Strategic Air Command and the Joint Strategic Target Planning Staff (the staff created to build the U.S. nuclear war plans) at Offutt Air Force Base were disestablished, and the U.S. Strategic Command was created. The United States signed START II with the Russian Federation in 1993, in which they agreed to

[3] In 1994 as part of the Budapest Memorandum, Ukraine gave up its Soviet nuclear weapons. In exchange, Ukrainian geopolitical borders were recognized and the country was to receive protection from the use of military force or economic sanctions by the Russian Federation, the United States, and the United Kingdom (*Memorandum on Security Assurances in Connection with Ukraine's Accession to the Treaty on Non-Proliferation of Nuclear Weapons*, Budapest, December 5, 1994).

eliminate all multiple-warhead land-based intercontinental ballistic missiles. Strategic exchange assessments indicated this would have been a major step forward for crisis stability, since in any attack on single-warhead intercontinental ballistic missiles, the attacker would be disarmed as rapidly as the victim, offering no advantage to a first nuclear strike. Unfortunately, however, the treaty never was implemented.

President Clinton was the first president to produce a Nuclear Posture Review (completed in 1994) to outline U.S. nuclear strategy. Given the scale of change in the global situation, it was perhaps surprising how much continuity there was in the review: the basic precepts of U.S. deterrent strategy remained largely unchanged. The review concluded that the United States should lead but hedge, meaning that it should pursue additional nuclear arms reductions but maintain the ability to return to higher levels of nuclear arms should circumstances change. Key elements of the U.S. nuclear strategy that remained unchanged included maintaining options for limited nuclear war fighting, focusing on counterforce targeting, preserving the option to use nuclear weapons first in a conflict, maintaining very high states of alert, preserving an option to launch missiles on warning of an attack, and maintaining nuclear weapons in Europe.

President Clinton pursued START III discussions with Russia, as well as a variety of initiatives related to monitoring nuclear weapon dismantlement and fissile material storage without revealing classified information. None of these initiatives fully came to fruition. Assessments of these initiatives focused mostly on the potential for long-term steps toward nuclear disarmament rather than how they might affect the probability or consequences of nuclear war.

In 1996, Clinton signed the Comprehensive Test Ban Treaty, but the U.S. Senate never ratified it despite administration assessments that the treaty would help slow nuclear proliferation, could be effectively verified, and would not prevent the United States from maintaining a safe and effective nuclear arsenal.

During this decade, the Nth-country problem again gained prominence. After the 1991 Gulf War, inspections revealed that Iraq had had a large nuclear weapons program, most of which had gone undetected. This led to reformed approaches to the International Atomic Energy Agency (IAEA) safeguards and to control of dual-use exports through the Nuclear Suppliers Group, an international group of nuclear supplier countries aiming to control proliferation through guidelines on nuclear exports.[4] Then, in 1994, a crisis over North Korea's nuclear program led to the Agreed Framework between the United States and North Korea in which North Korea agreed to freeze its plutonium program and allow international inspections in return for shipments of heavy fuel oil, steps toward diplomatic recognition, and construction of two light-water reactors.

[4] See the Nuclear Suppliers Group website at https://www.nuclearsuppliersgroup.org/en.

In 1995, the Nuclear Nonproliferation Treaty was extended indefinitely. But in 1998, both Pakistan and India carried out nuclear-explosion tests and formally declared themselves as nuclear-armed states, integrating nuclear weapons into their military forces. Meanwhile, with the collapse of the Soviet Union, nuclear theft and smuggling became a serious issue. The possibility of nuclear war occurring beyond the two superpowers—or of another nuclear state or terrorist group provoking a superpower nuclear conflict—began to appear of more concern.

The 2000s

Concerns about nuclear war risks in the 2000s were dominated by two factors: fears of nuclear attacks (or nuclear help to terrorists) by states the United States characterized as "rogue" states in Nuclear Posture Reviews, following the 9/11 attacks in 2001; and souring U.S.–Russian relations.

The George W. Bush administration, like the Clinton administration before it, undertook an overall review of the U.S. nuclear posture. It concluded that the United States needed a new triad that included its offensive nuclear forces, missile defenses, and a responsive infrastructure that would make it possible to build additional nuclear weapons, if needed (Frankel et al. 2016). The review also concluded that it was no longer necessary to size U.S. nuclear forces to match Russian forces; rather, U.S. forces should be large enough to cover the targets called for in U.S. nuclear strategy, regardless of whether Russian forces were larger or smaller.

Seeing potential threats from countries such as North Korea and Iran, the Bush administration accelerated U.S. missile defense plans and pulled out of the Anti-Ballistic Missile Treaty. In response, Russia decided not to implement START II (Arms Control Association 2001). Both sides, however, agreed to the Moscow Treaty, which used the framework and verification mechanisms of START and further reduced the numbers of nuclear weapons.

Extensive assessments were undertaken to examine how different types of missile defenses might address various future threats from North Korea and Iran. Few publicly available government analyses examined, however, the degree to which these same missile defenses might lead Russia and China to build larger offensive forces than would otherwise be the case, and what risks to U.S. security might result.

The dangers of multiple countries now maintaining nuclear arsenals began to garner attention and analysis. These assessments were based in significant part on concerns that accidents, false alarms, miscalculations, inadvertent escalation, and other unplanned events could lead to nuclear war, no matter what safety and security measures were in place.

The Agreed Framework collapsed during the 2000s, and North Korea carried out its first nuclear-explosion test in 2006. As North Korea continued to develop its nuclear forces, assessments focused both on verifying North Korean disarmament if agreement could be reached and on how to deter a nuclear-armed North Korea. These assessments focused primarily on intelligence assessments of North Korean capabilities and intent, technical assessments of the capabilities of U.S. offensive forces and missile defenses, and the use of expert judgment and wargaming to explore different deterrent strategies.

Also in the 2000s, Iran's secret nuclear efforts were revealed, provoking crises, sanctions, and on-again, off-again talks that ran throughout the decade. China's nuclear forces continued to expand during the decade but, despite growing Chinese capabilities, the United States did not acknowledge being in a mutual deterrence relationship with China.

Toward the end of the decade, President Barack Obama took power, with a very different vision of the future of nuclear weapons. In his Prague speech in 2009, he laid out a vision of a world free of nuclear weapons, as well as a series of steps he hoped to take to reduce nuclear dangers. He also noted, however, that nuclear disarmament might not be achieved in his lifetime and that the existence of nuclear weapons can serve as an effective nuclear deterrent.

The 2010s and Early 2020s

The Obama administration's 2010 Nuclear Posture Review, like previous reviews, assessed the adequacy of U.S. nuclear forces to carry out the deterrent missions assigned to them. This assessment involved strategic exchange calculations, technical assessments of the capability and reliability of particular weapon systems, intelligence assessments of adversary weapon systems, and expert judgments about what kinds of threats would deter what types of adversary actions. The assessment left most U.S. nuclear policies intact but indicated a strengthening of negative security assurance:

> The United States will not use or threaten to use nuclear weapons against non-nuclear weapons states that are party to the Nuclear Nonproliferation Treaty and in compliance with their nuclear nonproliferation obligations.... The United States affirms that any state eligible for the assurance that uses [chemical and biological weapons] against the United States or its allies and partners would face the prospect of a devastating conventional military response—and that any individuals responsible for the attack, whether national leaders or military commanders, would be held fully accountable. (OSD 2010)

Subsequently, the Obama administration laid out a 30-year $1.2 trillion plan to modernize all aspects of the U.S. nuclear arsenal, including additional safety and security enhancements. That plan was largely developed on the basis of engineering assessments of how long particular weapons in the existing arsenal would last and what would be needed to continue current U.S. nuclear strategies. The Trump administration generally endorsed the modernization program, while adding a low-yield submarine-launched ballistic missile warhead and plans for a nuclear sea-launched cruise missile. The Biden administration has so far mostly continued these previous plans, though the future of the nuclear sea-launched cruise missile is unclear.

The New START treaty was completed in 2010, reducing each side's deployed strategic forces to 1,550 warheads and 700 launchers. The treaty was subject to a variety of complex assessments: U.S. assessments confirmed that the treaty would be adequately verifiable, that U.S. forces within the limits would be sufficient to carry out their deterrent missions, and that the predictability and transparency offered by the treaty would help in planning U.S. strategic forces.

In the three-quarters of a century living with nuclear weapons, the United States has adopted a national security strategy that has strategic deterrence at its core (Bradley 2007; OSD 2018). As the committee heard in briefings from the U.S. Strategic Command, the United States views deterrence holistically, taking deterrence to refer to decisive influence on an adversary's decision-making calculus in order to prevent hostile action against vital interests. This view incorporates a recognition that deterrence must be tailored to the unique goals, values, and culture of specific adversaries.

This definition accounts for the likelihood that an adversary considers more than just the costs associated with an action they are contemplating. They compare the costs of a course of action to the benefits they seek, while also examining the consequences if they do not act. If an adversary believes that the costs associated with an action are credible and will be incurred, deterrence may still fail if the adversary perceives that the consequences of restraint are greater. This approach implies that deterrence strategies consider adversary perceptions of both the costs and benefits of a course of action, as well as their perceptions of the costs and benefits of restraint.

INSIGHTS RELEVANT TO THE RISKS OF NUCLEAR WAR

There are many complex ideas about risks associated with nuclear deterrence, both in theory and in practice. The literature is vast[5] but four ideas about nuclear risks have been especially influential, sometimes misunderstood, and sometimes ignored in practice: the reciprocal fear of surprise attack, the threat that leaves something to chance, the commitment trap, and the risk of inaction. They remain essential for proper understanding of nuclear risks.

[5] Important efforts to review this vast literature on nuclear deterrence theory and strategy include Freedman (2003) and Tetlock et al. (1989, 1991).

The Reciprocal Fear of Surprise Attack

Nuclear war between two states could be initiated out of "the dynamics of mutual alarm," even though neither planned nor desired to initiate a nuclear conflict (Schelling 1980, 2008). In this case, both governments prefer avoiding nuclear war, but both fear that the other might strike first and that the consequences of striking first are preferable to striking second. If war is deemed imminent and preemption is a preferred option, Schelling argued, each state might increase its nuclear alert level for the sake of deterrence, but each might also fear that such actions mean that the other was preparing for a surprise attack. Schelling's original model included a state placing extra (potentially less reliable) warning systems on alert as the fear of surprise attack increased. This would reduce the risk of a false confirmation that no attack was being launched (false negative) but increases the probability of a false warning of attack (false positive).

During the early Cold War, the Truman administration studied and then rejected the option of initiating a preventive war against the Soviet Union, but it maintained the option of launching a preemptive strike if a Soviet attack was deemed imminent and unavoidable (Truman and Lay 1950). However, because the United States could not be certain that it would receive accurate warning of an imminent Soviet attack and Cold War nuclear war plans, the administration's approach included both preemptive and retaliatory military options (Lynn 1969; Sagan 1987).

The dangers associated with mutual fears of preemption were highlighted during the 1962 Cuban missile crisis when a U.S. U-2 spy plane accidentally flew into Soviet airspace (Sagan 1993). Although neither the Russian nor the U.S. government has ever officially forsworn the option of a preemptive nuclear attack, both know that the other side's nuclear forces would largely survive an attack and both have invested heavily in redundant and (hopefully) independent and reliable warning systems.

But these mitigating factors may not exist in other conflict scenarios against new nuclear states. An example is the January 2018 incident in which a false warning of a North Korean missile attack was announced in Hawaii. The U.S. government did not overreact because redundant sensors reported that no attack was under way, professional warning system officers immediately reported that they had made a mistake, and U.S. officials did not believe that North Korea was likely to attack Hawaii. But it is instructive to imagine if this false warning incident had occurred in North Korea instead of the United States. None of the three mitigating factors would be as strong because North Korea's missile warning system is dependent on radars and has less redundancy, its officers might be less willing to acknowledge errors because the consequences of such acknowledgment could cost them more than just their livelihoods, and it could be perceived that a U.S. nuclear attack was likely given then-recent statements from President Donald Trump (Sagan 2018).

The Threat That Leaves Something to Chance

A threat that leaves something to chance is a strategy centered on making a credible threat of a nuclear first use in a situation that might otherwise be deemed unlikely to be implemented, such as responding to a conventional attack on an ally (Schelling 1960). Schelling provided two metaphors that helped illustrate the idea. First, while no individual could rationally threaten to jump off a cliff, the individual could rationally come closer and closer to the cliff and deliberately increase the chance of slipping off. Second, in the case of a fighter jet deliberately buzzing an adversary's fighter coming close to its border, the pilot was not threatening to deliberately crash into the enemy's plane; they were threatening to "accidentally" crash into it by losing control as they came closer. Such manipulation of risk was, Schelling argued, a core strategy of brinkmanship.

One application of this concept was the forward deployment of U.S. nuclear forces into NATO allies' territory. The idea was that such deployments would make extended deterrent commitments more credible even if a U.S. president might not want to use nuclear weapons in response to a conventional attack.

The danger of the threat that leaves something to chance is precisely that it leaves something to chance. Presidents since Kennedy have been reluctant to delegate nuclear launch authority to local commanders. After the Cuban missile crisis, locking devices were placed on U.S. nuclear weapons to reduce the risks of any unauthorized use of such weapons.

Delegation authority may exist in other nuclear states, however. Vipin Narang (2010, p. 87), for example, argues that in Pakistan, "lower-level officers may be ceded some authority, particularly as a crisis unfolds, to assemble and release Pakistani nuclear weapons should circumstances require it." This contributes, Narang argues, to an asymmetric escalation posture in which negative controls are "likely circumventable, by design, for deterrence purposes in a crisis or conflict situation with India" (Narang 2010, p. 90).

The Commitment Trap

The central idea of the commitment trap is that deterrent threats might not *reflect* existing commitments to use nuclear weapons, but rather *create* increased likelihood of nuclear use in the event of deterrence failure by linking the deterrent threat to a president's or the nation's reputation for honoring commitments (Sagan 2000). One example of this phenomenon occurred during the Cuban missile crisis. President Kennedy stated that the United States would act if Cuba should possess a capacity to carry out offensive action against the United States. He later believed that his earlier public warning boxed him into rejecting a diplomatic solution and into choosing a more serious military response (Bundy and Rosenblum 1989).

Experts hold a range of views about whether threats of nuclear response contributed to Saddam Hussein's decision not to use chemical or biological weapons in 1991. The U.S. Strategic Command's *Essentials of Post-Cold War Deterrence* report, for example, argues that this use of calculated ambiguity worked to deter Saddam Hussein (U.S. Strategic Command 1995). After examining the captured Iraqi records, however, independent scholars argued that Saddam Hussein never intended to use chemical weapons against U.S. troops on the battlefield; instead, he saw his chemical arsenal as a strategic deterrent to the United States and Israel nuclear threat (Buch and Sagan 2013).

The Risk of Inaction

The risk of inaction is poorly understood in much writing about deterrence. President Kennedy stated during the Cuban missile crisis that the risk of war with the Soviet Union was between one-third and one-half (Kennedy 1999). While President Kennedy's blockade of Cuba and threat of an attack if the Soviets did not remove the nuclear-armed missiles increased the risk of war, it is possible that the risks of a nuclear war might have been even greater in the future if the missiles remained in place. Not taking an action also entails risks.

THE HISTORY AND LITERATURE OF RISK ASSESSMENT FOR NUCLEAR TERRORISM

Risk assessments of nuclear and radiological terrorism have been conducted for many years, and the approaches and methods that have been used have evolved as threats of terrorism (and understanding of them) have changed. This overview includes a brief timeline of major events related to nuclear terrorism and the types of analyses that were produced to guide policy or decisions. While the literature presented in this report is U.S. centric, it is important to note that the literature from other countries and regions represents other historical experiences and strategic decisions.

Early Years (mid-1940s and 1950s)

Almost from the dawn of the nuclear age, there have been concerns over the possibility of covert emplacement of nuclear explosives.[6] In a 1946 congressional hearing, J. Robert Oppenheimer noted the feasibility that components of a nuclear bomb could be smuggled and then successfully detonated in a major city like New York. The Atomic Energy Commission (AEC)[7] then commissioned a study to assess detection capabilities against this threat (Lüth 2013; Richelson 2009). The threat of concern at that time was not of terrorist groups but of Soviet Union operatives placing such a bomb in a large city (Bunn et al. 2016; Zenko 2006).

Similarly, the first serious considerations of possible attacks on nuclear reactors focused on the possibility that national adversaries, such as communist countries, might attack them, not terrorist groups. For example, during the 1957 licensing process for the Turkey Point nuclear power reactor in Florida, opponents expressed concern that the reactor's proximity to Cuba would make it vulnerable to attack (Ramberg 1985; Travers 2001).

The 1960s

The concern about the origin of the threat shifted in the 1960s. A 1967 report to the AEC (Lumb et al. 1967) expressed concern that terrorists could acquire plutonium or highly enriched uranium and use these materials to make a crude nuclear bomb. The report recommended that safeguards and security programs "be designed in recognition of the problem of terrorist or criminal groups clandestinely acquiring nuclear weapons or materials useful therein" (Lumb et al. 1967, p. 331). The AEC responded with the first-ever rules requiring private owners of nuclear material to provide security for that material.

These early assessments of the risks and of the adequacy of security arrangements for nuclear weapons, materials, and facilities were largely based on expert judgment, not on systematic risk assessment approaches. Methods were largely speculative, based on imagining what adversaries might attempt to do and steps that could be taken to block those imagined pathways (Hirsch et al. 1986; Lumb et al. 1967; Ramberg 1985; Travers 2001).

---

[6] For summaries of portions of this history, see Bunn (2013), Bunn et al. (2016), Desmond et al. (1997), Richelson (2009), and Walker (2001).

[7] The AEC was responsible for designing and producing nuclear weapons, as well as encouraging the use of nuclear power and managing its safety regulations. The Energy Reorganization Act of 1974 transferred the regulatory functions of the AEC to the new Nuclear Regulatory Commission (NRC), and a few years later the Department of Energy was created to encourage the use of nuclear power and to manage the U.S. nuclear weapons.

The 1970s

By the 1970s, both public and government concern about the danger of nuclear terrorism had increased, driven by the rise of international terrorism following the 1967 Arab–Israeli war and increased threats to nuclear facilities. The 1972 attack at the Munich Olympics demonstrated that well-trained and well-armed terrorists could successfully carry out an assault in a modern developed country. Within the United States, hijackings and other terrorist-like incidents increased and were well publicized, including multiple nuclear threats and hoaxes (Bunn et al. 2016; Richelson 2009). Later, the Three Mile Island nuclear reactor accident in 1979 further focused the public's attention on nuclear risks.

The AEC commissioned an additional study of the adequacy of security arrangements, which concluded that existing security arrangements for nuclear material needed urgent improvement. Furthermore, the authors called for a design basis threat, which led to a new approach that is still in place today for assessing the adequacy of physical security measures at nuclear power facilities.[8]

These concerns provoked major changes in U.S. nuclear security requirements (Bunn 2013; Walker 2001). Still, others argued that terrorists would reject the level of violence that a nuclear attack would produce as it would not serve their political objectives (Bunn et al. 2016; JAEIC 1976).

During the 1970s, a variety of additional methods came into use for assessing aspects of the risks of nuclear terrorism and nuclear safety. The AEC and the new Nuclear Regulatory Commission (NRC) began applying systems engineering approaches to design and assess security systems in what came to be known as the design evaluation process overview. In 1975, the NRC issued the *Reactor Safety Study*, which was the first full-scale use of probabilistic risk assessment to quantify the risk of a nuclear reactor accident due to possible equipment and unintentional human failures. Assessments of the risk of sabotage of nuclear reactors also began to use insights from early probabilistic risk assessments.

The 1980s

The 1980s saw somewhat reduced public and government attention to the risks of nuclear terrorism and little change to the threat assessments of the 1970s. Cold War tensions in the early 1980s and the 1986 Chernobyl nuclear accident focused attention instead on the dangers of nuclear war and on nuclear accidents.

[8] Earlier, the WASH-740 report (AEC 1957) had identified major uncertainties in the scientific knowledge basis for evaluating the consequences of major nuclear reactor accidents. Coincidentally, in 1975 the *Reactor Safety Study* (known as WASH-1400 [NRC 1975]) used risk assessment methods for the first time to estimate the risks of an accidental exposure to members of the public due to a nuclear power station accident.

Nevertheless, congressional investigations of security for U.S. nuclear facilities continued, the executive branch remained concerned because of both security failures at U.S. facilities and continuing terrorist attacks around the world, and some private analysts remained quite concerned (Leventhal and Alexander 1987).

The 1986 national intelligence estimate, *The Likelihood of Nuclear Acts by Terrorist Groups*, concluded, as had the 1976 and 1977, that a few terrorist groups were capable of making a nuclear bomb but behavioral constraints made it unlikely (Director of Central Intelligence 1986). This view of the problem, which was reached largely through analysis of the historical record and of imputed terrorist incentives, held for much of the next decade and a half.

The 1990s

The collapse of the Soviet Union in 1991, and the social, political, and economic disruptions that followed, led to problems with security for nuclear weapons, materials, and facilities in the former Soviet states. There were multiple well-documented thefts of kilogram quantities of highly enriched uranium or separated plutonium. U.S. intelligence concluded that nuclear facilities in the former Soviet Union did not have adequate safeguards and security (Allison et al. 1996; Bukharin 1996; Bunn 2000).

Concerns over "loose nukes" were exacerbated by increasingly violent terrorist actions. In Japan, the terror cult Aum Shinrikyo, which carried out nerve gas attacks in the Tokyo subway system, had also pursued both nuclear and biological weapons. Osama bin Laden's al-Qaeda group bombed the U.S. embassies in Kenya and Tanzania in 1998, sought nuclear weapons, and announced that it was their religious duty to acquire weapons of mass destruction (Daly et al. 2005; Danzig et al. 2012).

The United States responded with counterterrorist efforts against al-Qaeda and other groups, and a program to help secure nuclear weapons and materials in the former Soviet states (National Research Council 1999, 2009).

The 2000s and Beyond

The 2000s and beyond saw further shifts in terrorist threats, nuclear security, and refinements of assessment methods. Assessments of the threat of nuclear and radiological terrorism were fundamentally transformed by the 9/11 attacks in the United States. These attacks demonstrated that some terrorist groups were, in fact, seeking to cause catastrophic loss of life. Moreover, they showed that coordinated attacks involving multiple trained teams, prior collection of intelligence and specialized training, and a willingness to die as part of the plan were realistic threats

(Ezel et al. 2010; Merrick and Parnell 2011; Parnell et al. 2011; Rosoff and von Winterfeldt 2007; Willis et al. 2005).

Investigations after the 2001 attacks revealed far more about al-Qaeda's nuclear, radiological, chemical, and biological efforts than had previously been known. Terrorists working with al-Qaeda also considered attacks on nuclear reactors and the use of radiological dispersal devices, though the unclassified literature does not make clear how far those efforts proceeded (Mowatt-Larssen and Allison 2010; Tenet 2007). In addition, North Caucasus terrorists (Chechens and others) reportedly pursued nuclear or radiological weapons, according to the Russian state newspaper, *Rossiskaya Gazeta*, which also separately reported additional cases of terrorist reconnaissance on nuclear weapon transport trains.

In response, the U.S. government increased security requirements for both government and commercial nuclear facilities, as did a number of other countries (GAO 2004a,b). The United States implemented changes to further protect nuclear facilities, including nuclear weapons storage/handling sites under the Department of Defense, nuclear weapons complex facilities run by the Department of Energy, and commercial nuclear facilities licensed and regulated by the NRC. Box 3-1 provides a description of NRC-regulated security requirements for commercial nuclear facilities; the Department of Defense and the Department of Energy have similar security requirements and protocols in place for their respective facilities that handle nuclear weapons and nuclear materials.

BOX 3-1
Physical Security Requirements for Nuclear Facilities

The Nuclear Regulatory Commission (NRC) security orders for commercial nuclear power reactor licensees and Category I Fuel Cycle Facilities[a] aim to ensure security through the concept of the design basis threat. This approach provides a general description of the attributes of potential adversaries who might attempt to commit radiological sabotage or theft or diversion of special nuclear material against which the licensee's physical protection systems must defend with high assurance (10 CFR § 73).[b] The design basis threat incorporates a number of security concepts, including insider threats, cyber vulnerability, potential attacks by multiple coordinated teams, suicide attacks, and air- or waterborne threats.

In order to test the adequacy of facilities' protective strategies, the NRC conducts periodic performance-based inspections (called force-on-force exercises) to assess the ability of the security systems (e.g., physical fences, motion detectors, alarms, armed guards) to counter the design basis threat (NRC 2019).

[a] The NRC classifies facilities that possess special nuclear materials into three categories according to the materials' potential for use in nuclear weapons (i.e., their strategic significance). Category I refers to facilities with high strategic significance.

[b] See 10 CFR § 73.1 for a list of design basis threats. See 10 CFR §§ 73.20, 73.45, and 73.46 for general performance objectives and capabilities for fixed site physical protection systems.

During the 2000s, the government also created the Department of Homeland Security (through the Homeland Security Act, P.L. 107-296) in 2002 and the Domestic Nuclear Detection Office in 2005 to coordinate U.S. federal efforts to detect and protect against nuclear and radiological terrorism) (DHS 2021; Gaertner and Teagarden 2006; Helfand et al. 2002).[9]

The heightened concern also led to a flurry of international activity related to preventing nuclear terrorism. The IAEA launched a new nuclear security fund to finance expanded IAEA nuclear security programs. In 2002, less than a year after the 9/11 attacks, the leaders of what was then the Group of Eight launched the Global Partnership Against the Spread of Weapons and Materials of Mass Destruction, in which the participants pledged to invest $20 billion over 10 years in cooperative activities for threat reduction activities (NTI 2002). In 2004, the United Nations (UN) Security Council unanimously passed Resolution 1540, which legally obligated all member states to criminalize any help to terrorists with weapons of mass destruction and to create security and accounting for any nuclear, chemical, or biological weapons or materials those states might have (UN Security Council 2004). In 2005, an amendment was made to the UN physical protection convention to extend the convention's coverage from civilian nuclear material in international transport to civilian material in domestic use and to include sabotage. The convention entered into force in 2016.[10] The same year, the Russian-proposed International Convention on the Suppression of Acts of Nuclear Terrorism was opened for signature (Perera 2005). In 2006, Russia and the United States jointly launched the Global Initiative to Combat Nuclear Terrorism (DOS 2009; National Research Council 2002).

After the deaths of key al-Qaeda leaders, including Osama bin Laden in May 2011, the United States determined al-Qaeda's capability to launch catastrophic attacks on the United States to have been substantially reduced (Office of the Coordinator for Counterterrorism 2012). Nevertheless, al-Qaeda operations continued and still continue in a number of countries, and many of the identified participants in al-Qaeda's nuclear effort remain at large. Moreover, the violent jihadist movement continues to spread. The Islamic State, originally an off-shoot of al-Qaeda, is an important example of a rapidly evolving threat: it was not mentioned in the 2014 U.S. intelligence community's annual assessment of threats to the country. But by June 2014, the group had seized much of Iraq and Syria and declared a global caliphate. While the Islamic State's geographic caliphate has since been destroyed,

[9] In 2018 the Domestic Nuclear Detection Office was combined with the Office of Health Affairs into the Countering Weapons of Mass Destruction Office.

[10] See International Atomic Energy Agency, "Convention on the Physical Protection of Nuclear Material (CPPNM) and its Amendment," https://www.iaea.org/publications/documents/conventions/convention-physical-protection-nuclear-material-and-its-amendment.

the group continues to have followers operating in many countries, and it still has access to substantial resources.

Between 2010 and 2016, efforts to strengthen nuclear security around the world accelerated with a series of global nuclear security summits, which helped focus attention and accelerate various actions, such as removal of nuclear material from vulnerable sites (Cann et al. 2016). However, U.S.–Russian cooperation on nuclear security was almost entirely terminated after Russia's 2014 annexation of Crimea (then part of Ukraine), leaving little remaining communication between the countries with the world's two largest nuclear complexes (Bunn and Kovchegin 2018).

During this period, methods for assessing aspects of the risks of nuclear and radiological terrorism progressed slowly. There were enhanced efforts to model the economic and social effects of a nuclear or radiological attack, using both economic models and agent-based modeling (Chandan et al. 2013; Vargas 2020; Vargas and Ehlen 2013), as well as efforts to model and test the performance of nuclear security systems in the face of intelligent adversaries. The Department of Homeland Security and Domestic Nuclear Detection Office explored risk analysis to guide decisions (Streetman 2011), but most of the methods pursued were refinements of methods already applied in the 2000s.

The Fukushima Phase 2 report (NASEM 2016) allowed that adversarial intent could be included in risk assessments. This was a notable shift from earlier consensus reports from the National Academies of Sciences, Engineering, and Medicine, which had largely concluded that modeling adversarial intent using such risk assessment methods as probabilistic risk assessment was not feasible (National Research Council 2006, 2011, 2013).

One new assessment effort was the Nuclear Threat Initiative's Nuclear Security Index, published every 2 years starting in 2012.[11] The index uses a variety of indicators of the status of areas, ranging from security and control measures at individual sites to risk environment, to give an overall rating on how countries are doing on nuclear security. The countries' ratings determine their ranking.

The International Picture

Since the 2001 terrorist attacks in the United States, some other governments have shared a substantial level of concern about nuclear terrorism. For example, Norway (Karamoskos 2009), Canada (Etchegary et al. 2008), and Australia (Gaidow 2007; Hirst 2007) have explored public perceptions of the risks and the impact of the 9/11 attacks to national security. Counterterrorism activities and efforts to improve security for nuclear weapons, materials, and facilities and to stop nuclear smuggling have been global initiatives.

[11] For more information, see the NTI Nuclear Security Index website at https://www.ntiindex.org.

Russia, in particular, made efforts to reduce the threat of nuclear terrorism. The country first proposed the nuclear terrorism convention, and they joined with the United States in launching the Global Initiative to Combat Nuclear Terrorism in 2006. These programs have worked to improve how detection of material out of regulatory control is communicated and addressed among law enforcement agencies and governments and to test physical security measures and responses to possible terrorist events.

IAEA efforts that focused on nuclear security expanded dramatically after the 9/11 attacks. IAEA's small Office of Physical Protection became the Office of Nuclear Security, which has now become the Division of Nuclear Security, funded at tens of millions of dollars a year. IAEA expanded its review services, launched a nuclear security series of documents, greatly expanded its training programs in nuclear security, and increased its efforts to collect and analyze various types of data, from incidents to program implementations. In particular, IAEA now offers guidance on assessment methodologies for physical protection of nuclear facilities and implementation of radiation detection to counter nuclear smuggling. However, there is no international agreement on methods for assessing the threat of nuclear and radiological terrorism.

INSIGHTS RELEVANT TO THE RISKS OF NUCLEAR TERRORISM

As with nuclear war, there are fortunately few data on actual cases of nuclear terrorism to draw from. Nevertheless, there is a great deal of data on terrorism more generally, and some data on past terrorist attempts to acquire nuclear weapons, make radiological dispersal devices, or sabotage nuclear facilities. These three categories of activity involve different levels of violence and immediate effect, have different levels of technological complexity, and may have different theoretical implications. The discussion below focuses primarily on the most extreme form of nuclear or radiological terrorism: the actual use of nuclear explosives.

Several key insights relevant to assessing the risks of nuclear terrorism have been drawn from the broader set of data on terrorist activities over the decades. These insights relate to terrorist motivation, technical ambition and capability; the factors affecting the availability of nuclear weapons and materials; and the chances that states might choose to help terrorists get nuclear explosives. Although experience and the theoretical literature help explore kinds of groups that may be interested in nuclear violence, terrorist groups are varied and ever changing. The following insights should be considered tendencies and not absolute rules.

Terrorist Motivations: No Longer Just "A Lot of People Watching"

The understanding of terrorist motivations has evolved over recent decades. Analysts exploring the motivations of different terrorist groups have identified the following types of groups that may be inclined toward mass slaughter (Ferguson et al. 2005):

- Nihilist groups, interested in destruction for its own sake;
- Millennial groups, who envision the end of the world and want to help hasten it (such as Aum Shinrikyo); and
- Groups with extreme objectives, such as taking down a superpower or achieving world domination, for which weapons of extraordinary power might seem appropriate (such as al-Qaeda and the Islamic State).

Many advanced democracies are coping with increasing right-wing extremism. Some of these groups and individuals appear to fall into the "extreme objectives" category and have been focused on nuclear themes. *The Turner Diaries*, a novel that is a foundational text for racist extremists in the United States, envisions using nuclear weapons against U.S. cities to bring down the prevailing multiracial society and establish a white supremacist state. The manifesto written by Anders Breivik, the terrorist who massacred students and bombed the parliament in Norway, explores nuclear themes at length, including a detailed discussion of sabotaging nuclear facilities. One neo-Nazi extremist group in the United States even named itself the "Atomwaffen Division" (see, e.g., Earnhardt et al. 2021).

Deterring Terrorists and Terrorist Deterrence

Although it is not obvious that a terrorist group that acquired a nuclear bomb would immediately choose to use it (Dunn 2005), history makes clear that terrorist groups are difficult to deter. However, many types of terrorist groups can be, and have been, deterred from taking some types of terrorist actions. When groups have territory and populations they control, or for whom they are fighting, they may be motivated to avoid actions that could provoke retaliation on those populations. Some analysts have argued that if terrorists did get a nuclear bomb, it would serve their interests better not to detonate it, but to hold it to deter attacks against them. In a 1999 interview, Osama bin Laden claimed that al-Qaeda had nuclear and chemical weapons as a deterrent that it would use in retaliation for nuclear or chemical attacks against Muslims (Dunn 2005). However, the existence of such terrorist weapons would likely provoke a global effort to find and eliminate them.

Terrorist Technical Ambitions: "Sticking with the Tried and True"

Another relevant set of analyses has focused on the weapons terrorists use. The overwhelming majority of terrorist groups focus on conventional weapons. Recently, some terrorist attacks have been even simpler, using vans or cars driven into crowds, for example. Analysts have noted that terrorists, facing the constant possibility of being caught, typically want to carry out actions with a high chance of success—or at least of getting far enough to be very visible and provoke fear (Jenkins 2008). Using challenging new types of weapons that may take a long period to figure out and may not work have not typically been something most terrorist groups have pursued.

Nevertheless, some terrorist groups have actively attempted to develop nuclear, biological, and chemical weapons, including Aum Shinrikyo and al-Qaeda. There is little publicly available evidence of a focused nuclear weapons effort by the Islamic State, but it did manufacture and use its own chemical and conventional weapons and carry out a rapid program of testing and improving its drones for bomb delivery (see, e.g., Gartenstein-Ross et al. 2019; Tønnessen 2017).

Making nuclear explosives requires not only the factual knowledge that can be conveyed in written documents, but the tacit knowledge that comes only with prior experience. Because terrorist groups will not typically have anyone with prior experience making nuclear weapons, it is argued, they would have difficulty producing a nuclear bomb (Ouagrham-Gormley 2007). But it should be recalled that repeated government studies have concluded that it is plausible that a sophisticated terrorist group could make a crude nuclear bomb; in the case of highly enriched uranium, the technical requirements are straightforward; and states have almost always succeeded in their very first nuclear test, even when they had no personnel with prior tacit knowledge available to help.

Terrorist Capabilities for Complex, Long-Term Projects: "The Terrorist's Dilemma"

Many terrorist groups have had trouble organizing complex, long-term projects in part because of the constant possibility of being interrupted by counterterrorism forces. Shapiro (2013) identified the terrorist's dilemma: on one hand, in order to maximize their perceived chance of accomplishing their group's objectives, leaders of a terrorist group need to communicate with their operatives and convince them to carry out the activities the leadership thinks will contribute to the cause and avoid the activities the leadership thinks will undermine the cause; on the other hand, all communications and gatherings of leadership and operatives increase the chance of being detected and stopped by counterterrorism forces. Terrorist leaders,

Shapiro argues, must constantly balance these concerns, and this constrains how terrorist organizations are managed.

In most cases, a nuclear bomb project would require recruiting technical experts and weeks, months, or years of work. The leadership of the group may not need to get involved in day-to-day management of the effort, but it likely needs to provide resources and keep the people motivated and working overtime. Thus, such efforts might well run up against the kind of dilemma Shapiro identified.

CONCLUSION

CONCLUSION 3-1: The U.S. nuclear posture has evolved over time, taking into account new threats, developing deterrence strategies against different U.S. adversaries, technological advancements, nuclear arms reductions, and changing geopolitical environments. U.S. assessments of the risks of nuclear terrorism have likewise evolved over time, taking into account the new threats and emerging technologies.

4

The Use of Risk Assessment for Nuclear War and Nuclear Terrorism

The threats of nuclear war and terrorism have evolved over the years as the geopolitical landscape and the leadership, capabilities, and objectives of U.S. adversaries have changed. The nuclear capabilities of the United States have also evolved. This chapter offers a snapshot of some of the current threats contributing to the risks of nuclear war or terrorism and a discussion of what is known about the range of possible consequences of nuclear war and nuclear terrorism.

THREATS OF NUCLEAR WAR

Though the world's stockpile of nuclear weapons has been reduced by more than 80 percent since its Cold War peak, unclassified estimates suggest that some 13,000 nuclear weapons remain in the world. Clearly, numbers alone do not tell the whole story: for instance, the role of new weapons and technologies has become increasingly significant. Yet, as the destruction of Hiroshima and Nagasaki showed in 1945, one nuclear weapon can instantly destroy much of a city and kill tens or hundreds of thousands of people. Much has changed since then, in world politics, in technology, and in nuclear policies—including, not least, the collapse of the Soviet Union, the end of the global Cold War, the acknowledgment of a larger number of nuclear states, and the emergence of other technologies (e.g., hypersonic weapons, cyber capabilities, artificial intelligence, and disinformation).

While no nuclear weapons have been detonated in conflict since 1945, the risk of nuclear war and nuclear and radiological terrorism remains very real. The challenge presented to this committee is how one might assess those risks. In an analytical process, a risk analyst would begin by identifying the risks associated with nuclear war and nuclear terrorism, describing classes of scenarios that involve either nuclear war or nuclear terrorism. The next steps would include exploring what is known about the probabilities of their occurrence, the uncertainties, other military and nonmilitary options, and the possible consequences of the use of nuclear weapons. This section explores those factors.

The scenarios of potential future nuclear conflicts considered here happen in the context of a roughly 10-year time horizon. Key questions include the following: How will these open or latent conflicts evolve? What scenarios could lead to different directions? How can risk analysis shed some light on various risk reduction options?

The committee does not attempt to assess the magnitude of the risks of nuclear war posed at this time by these different conflicts. The order in which the issues are discussed below is based on the total number of nuclear weapons that could potentially be targeted on the United States.

The United States and Russia

The United States and Russia possess approximately 90 percent of the known nuclear weapons in the world. Tensions between the two countries are high as this report is being written, having taken a severe downturn after Russia's annexation of Crimea in 2014 and the U.S. and European imposition of sanctions in response. These tensions have been exacerbated by Russia's 2022 invasion of Ukraine, during which Russia has threatened the use of nuclear weapons.

Former senator Sam Nunn and former Secretary of Energy Ernest Moniz argued in 2019 that this geopolitical hostility, the cutoff of various forms of communication and cooperation, and evolving technologies may undermine the stability of deterrent balances (Moniz and Nunn 2019). Because of ongoing hostility between the two sides, nearly all military-to-military contact below the highest levels, nearly all legislator-to-legislator contact, and nearly all contact between nuclear scientists has been ended. As of 2022, the world's two largest nuclear complexes are modernizing and developing new weapon systems, increasing some of their arsenals' capabilities, and proceeding in virtually total isolation from each other. One particularly worrisome scenario involves Russia's attempt to reestablish control over the Baltic states, which could start with a fast-paced conventional invasion followed by a limited nuclear attack intended to consolidate military gains and prompt the North Atlantic Trade Organization to come to the negotiating table rather than countering Russia's advances directly.

The United States and China

Tensions between the United States and China have also risen dramatically in recent years. China's economic and military power has grown, and China's foreign policy has become more assertive. As with Russia, China and the United States each have a long list of complaints about the other's behavior.

China possesses hundreds of nuclear weapons, compared with the thousands in the U.S. and Russian nuclear arsenals, but a major modernization of its nuclear forces is under way. As of early 2021, the U.S. intelligence community expected China to at least double the size of its nuclear stockpile over the next decade (ODNI 2021). Nongovernment analysts have also noted that China appears to be building hundreds of new silos for what may be intercontinental ballistic missiles (Korda and Kristensen 2021).

China has declared a policy of no-first-use of nuclear weapons and contends that this greatly reduces the risks of nuclear conflict. But it is easy to imagine scenarios in which a regional conflict might escalate to higher levels of violence, such as a Chinese attempt to force Taiwan reunification (Talmadge 2017). Chinese conventionally armed missiles would pose a serious threat to U.S. naval forces in such a conflict, possibly leading to a U.S. decision to attempt to destroy many of these missiles. But as China, like other countries, has missiles and command systems with dual nuclear and conventional roles, such a U.S. attack might be seen as the beginning of an effort to destroy China's nuclear forces, calling for a nuclear response. This mixing of nuclear and conventional forces (which exists in most nuclear states) has come to be known as entanglement and could increase the risks of escalation that neither side initially intended (Acton 2018). Some U.S. analysts argue that China is overconfident in its ability to control escalation, potentially increasing risks (Cunningham and Fravel 2019).

China has not participated in nuclear arms control, so there are no treaties or political commitments limiting its nuclear forces, except for (1) the broad Nuclear Nonproliferation Treaty obligation to negotiate in good faith toward both general and nuclear disarmament and (2) the Comprehensive Nuclear Test Ban Treaty, which—like the United States—it has signed but not ratified. Moreover, as of late 2021, there were no strategic stability talks under way between the United States and China, and there were few confidence-building measures, such as notification of missile launches or military-to-military cooperation.

The United States and North Korea

It is estimated that North Korea now has dozens of nuclear weapons and a variety of missiles to deliver them. It has tested missiles with the range and payload necessary to reach nearly all of the continental United States. While it has not carried out full-scale tests of reentry vehicles at that range, it is probably safest to assume that North Korea could deliver nuclear weapons to the United States; and it could, with greater certainty, threaten South Korea, Japan, and China.

The Kim family dictatorship that rules North Korea has long shown a savvy instinct for survival—illustrating how deterrence can be effective. They have a history of violent provocations against South Korea, such as the 2010 shelling of a South Korean island and the sinking of a South Korean ship in the same year. In the future, one could easily imagine another such provocation escalating to large-scale conflict, which could lead North Korea to believe its survival depended on disabling South Korean and U.S. attacks by using nuclear weapons. In such a conflict, North Korea might use a small number of conventionally armed missiles against U.S. and South Korean air bases to interfere with joint air operations. Once North Korea had begun firing its missiles, the United States and South Korea might launch an air campaign to destroy the remaining North Korean missiles before they could do more damage. That air campaign would create pressure on the North to use its nuclear weapons before they were destroyed; the air campaign might be seen by the North as preparation for an all-out invasion that had to be stopped by destroying key U.S. bases with nuclear weapons. That initial use might then lead to a larger-scale nuclear conflict.[1]

India and Pakistan

India and Pakistan are each thought to have more 100 nuclear weapons, as well as a range of systems to deliver them. The relative proximity of each country to the other may complicate effective early warning. Neither is likely to attack the United States, but nuclear war between the two of them is believed to be quite possible. The two have fought four wars since independence; they share a hotly disputed border; and they have hostile relations, little communication, and few agreements or confidence-building measures to help manage their conflict. A 2019 clash led to the interception of an Indian military aircraft over Pakistan and heated public calls for war on both sides. In addition, a technical malfunction during maintenance in March 2022 launched an Indian missile into Pakistan and reignited the debate on risk mitigation and nuclear weapon responsibility in the region (Shahzad et al. 2022).

India and Pakistan's respective military and nuclear doctrines—if implemented as each side threatens—could lead directly to nuclear war and potentially draw in other nuclear powers, such as Russia or the United States, into an escalated global war. India, seeking to deter Pakistan from sponsoring terrorist attacks, could posture its conventional forces to pose a threat such that an attack could lead to a rapid

[1] For a plausible scenario of how a U.S.-North Korean nuclear war might begin, see Lewis (2018).

Indian incursion into Pakistani territory. Pakistan, seeking to deter such an Indian invasion, could threaten to use tactical nuclear weapons to stop Indian forces from entering Pakistan. India, seeking to deter Pakistan from using nuclear weapons, could reinforce warnings that if Pakistan uses any nuclear weapons, the war will not remain limited and India will launch full strategic nuclear strikes against Pakistani targets. This could result in a full Pakistani retaliation with whatever forces survived the Indian strike.

Recently, some Indian officials have suggested that India might not wait for such a series of events, but might try to attack Pakistani nuclear weapons and destroy them before they could be used.

THREATS OF NUCLEAR TERRORISM

As discussed in the historical review of the literature on assessment methods for nuclear terrorism in Chapter 3, the U.S. approach toward nuclear terrorism threats has evolved with the threats: from a limited focus on clandestine actions by the Soviet Union to terrorist groups with motivations to inflict great harm to a large number of people. A consistent theme across decades of analysis is that it is the difficulty in obtaining nuclear material that remains one the most effective means of preventing nuclear terrorism. While much work has been done over the past decades to successfully secure nuclear materials, threats of nuclear terrorism still remain.

To understand the extent of the current possibilities for nuclear terrorism, one must consider terrorists' motives, capabilities, and opportunities. For motive, there is an enduring goal for a variety of terrorist groups to inflict great harm on the United States, its population, and allies. Capabilities of a terrorist group can change rapidly, either with acquisition of nuclear materials or devices, or with sudden surges in influence. Finally, opportunities to obtain nuclear materials persist as some materials are not well secured, and insider threats remain real (Bunn 2021).

Evidence collected from terrorist groups indicates that there is interest in developing and using improvised nuclear devices and radiological dispersal devices (Bunn et al. 2019). As noted in Chapter 3, for example, the Japanese terror cult Aum Shinikyo conducted nerve gas attacks in Matsumoto in 1994 and in Tokyo subways in 1995 and had previously focused efforts to get nuclear and biological weapons. Core al-Qaeda pursued nuclear weapons, carried out conventional explosive tests, and considered attacks on nuclear reactors, and their affiliates pursued radioactive material for a radiological dispersal device. Chechen terrorists planted a dangerous radiological source in a Moscow park as a warning, threatened to use radiological dispersal devices, and repeatedly threatened and planned attacks on reactors. In addition, Russian officials have reported catching terrorist teams scoping nuclear weapon storage sites and transports.

Current understanding of terrorism threats will continue to change as the United States and others continue to address the problem, and as adversaries react to those improvements. Risk analysis is one way to identify what components of the problem may be addressable.

Contributors to Nuclear Material Availability

It is challenging for terrorist groups, as they exist today, to produce their own plutonium or highly enriched uranium. To achieve nuclear weapons capability, they would likely have to secure a state-made nuclear weapon and figure out how to detonate it, or get plutonium or highly enriched uranium and figure out how to make a crude nuclear bomb of their own. Hence, ensuring that nuclear weapons and weapons-usable nuclear material are protected from theft, and blocking smuggling of any nuclear material that is outside of state control, remain critical to preventing nuclear terrorism. Similarly, ensuring effective security for major nuclear facilities and for radiological materials is important for reducing the dangers of those types of terrorism.

As discussed in Chapter 3, the problem of security for nuclear weapons or materials came to widespread attention in the 1970s, and what were loosely termed "loose nukes" became an even greater concern after the collapse of the Soviet Union in 1991.

How states and organizations managing these materials decide what types of security measures to implement and how much is enough is still not well understood. The results of such decisions vary widely, from states that do not require *any* armed guards at nuclear facilities to states that require on-site armed protection capable of fighting off a substantial force of attackers. These decisions are not necessarily correlated with resources and experience. It often takes a major incident to drive improvements in nuclear security arrangements, but responses to such incidents are modulated by the particular regulatory arrangements and organizational cultures of different countries.[2] Many efforts—ranging from bilateral technical cooperation to recommendations and review and training programs of the International Atomic Energy Agency (IAEA) to the nuclear security summits of 2010–2016—have strengthened nuclear security around the world and eliminated weapons-usable nuclear material entirely from many countries. However, much remains to be done, and the underlying factors that lead states to adopt and maintain stringent nuclear security measures remain mysterious.

Two of the most important and difficult nuclear security challenges are coping with an insider threat and maintaining strong security cultures. All the cases of theft of highly enriched uranium or plutonium (where enough is known about the

[2] For an initial attempt at collecting data in this area, see Bunn and Harrell (2014).

incident to know how it happened) were perpetrated by known and trusted insiders at the facility, or with the help of insiders. The same is true of most of the known cases of attempted sabotage of nuclear power plants. But insider threats are difficult to cope with: insiders have authorized access to go through many of the layers of a facility's security system; they may understand the facility's security system and its weaknesses; and a variety of cognitive and organizational biases often lead organizations not to suspect these insiders until it is too late (Bunn and Sagan 2017). The growing problem of violent nationalist extremists in advanced democracies may increase the insider threat. More work is still needed to understand how best to address insider threats without undermining the cooperation and trust essential for organizations to do their work.

Security culture—the degree to which all personnel take security seriously and are constantly on the lookout for threats that need to be addressed or for weaknesses that need to be corrected—remains a critical and difficult problem. The best security technology will not provide effective security if the people in the security system are not paying adequate attention. In 2012, for example, an 82-year-old nun and two other protestors went through three layers of alarmed fencing at the Y-12 nuclear site in Oak Ridge, Tennessee, and reached the building where thousands of bombs' worth of highly enriched uranium is stored. They pounded on the building with sledgehammers, sang peace songs, and poured blood and paint on the building before finally being accosted by a single guard. It turned out that the site had been directed to install a new alarm system and had tried to save money by combining it with the old system; the result had been some 10 times as many false alarms as before. There was, in short, a profound breakdown of security culture at one of the most secure sites in one of the countries with the most experience implementing nuclear security and some of the world's most stringent nuclear security rules. Many nuclear organizations around the world are attempting to strengthen nuclear security culture, but keeping people constantly on alert for threats that almost never occur is a major challenge (see, e.g., WINS 2016).

Social science theory and past experience related to black markets have provided important insights about potential nuclear black markets.[3] But while markets for items such as illicit drugs involve thousands of transactions taking place over years, with both criminals and law enforcement having the opportunity to observe each other and learn over time about what works and what does not, a seller with weapons-usable nuclear material continues to be a rare event, as is a real buyer.

How states decide how much effort to put behind steps to block nuclear smuggling—for example, implementing effective laws, creating dedicated police or intelligence teams trained and equipped to handle such cases, proactively organizing

[3] For a good summary of what is known about smuggling of stolen highly enriched uranium and plutonium, see Zaitseva and Steinhäusler (2014).

investigations and sting operations, or putting radiation detectors at key locations—remains another area of uncertainty, as is how to maintain strong security cultures and avoid insider threats in these areas.

Efforts to counter nuclear smuggling, too, vary widely among countries. Efforts such as the Global Initiative to Combat Nuclear Terrorism, the nuclear security summits, bilateral cooperation, and IAEA programs have helped eliminate some of the weakest points in the global system, but there is a great deal more to be done, and only modest understanding of the factors that are most important in determining state decisions.

Understanding Whether States Will Help with Nuclear Terrorism

There is a question of whether states would help terrorists get nuclear weapons, either for money or to carry out attacks for which a state hoped to avoid blame (Butler 2001). Some analysts consider the possibility that a country like North Korea (or Iran, were it to acquire nuclear weapons) might provide nuclear materials or weapons to terrorists to be a major part of the nuclear terrorism risks (Allison 2004). The fear that Saddam Hussein's Iraq might have been helping terrorists with nuclear, chemical, or biological weapons was one of the key public arguments for the U.S.-led invasion of Iraq in 2003 (Blitzer 2003).

Others argue that conscious state decisions to help terrorists with nuclear weapons are extremely unlikely and probably only a small part of the overall nuclear terrorism risks. The argument is that any such help would carry an enormous risk of being discovered, and dictators attempting to control everything in their states are unlikely to give the greatest power they have ever acquired to terrorist groups who might use it in ways that could provoke retaliation that would remove them from power. In that sense, there is a very big difference between selling a nuclear weapons capability to another state (such as North Korea's plutonium reactor export to Syria, which was ultimately destroyed by Israel) and providing such a capability to a terrorist group. While a wealthy terrorist group might be willing to offer substantial sums for such a capability, it is highly unlikely that terrorists would be able to provide enough money for the effect to be that the transaction would increase, rather than decrease, the chance of regime survival (Bunn 2006; Lieber and Press 2013).

CONSEQUENCES OF NUCLEAR AND RADIOLOGICAL WEAPONS USE

The consequences of nuclear war and terrorism can be described across several different dimensions, including the device or event type, the scale of the event, and the timelines and magnitude of the effects.

Timelines and Magnitude of Effect

The magnitude of the effects of the use of a nuclear or radiological weapon varies according to the time elapsed since the event occurred. The immediate effects of a nuclear explosion include an intense burst of gamma and neutron radiation; a fireball (anything inside the fireball is likely to be totally consumed); an intense, blinding flash and a pulse of thermal radiation (causing burns and igniting fires); a powerful blast wave, accompanied by intense winds; and an intense electromagnetic pulse (localized for blasts within the atmosphere, but more far-reaching for blasts in space).

Near- and long-term effects are wide reaching. In the near term (roughly, 1 hour to 1 week after the event), widespread evacuations and grid instability are possible along with initial radiation effects on humans. In the long term (weeks to several months or years after the event), effects include social and economic unrest, political and governance crises, health effects, infrastructure failures, negative environmental and climate effects, migration, and psychological distress (Glasstone and Dolan 1977; Jervis 1988; Katz and Osdoby 1982).

Radiological Dispersal Devices and Nuclear Sabotage

Nuclear or radiological terrorism could take several forms with different consequences. Recent studies have explored the consequences of various types of nuclear terrorism. Bunn and colleagues (2019) outline three types of nuclear terrorist events: improvised nuclear devices, radiological dispersal devices, and sabotage of nuclear facilities. They found that the latter two types have similar consequences that are smaller in magnitude than the consequences from improvised nuclear devices. Another study explored the effects of a single terrorist nuclear bomb (Bunn and Roth 2017). Effects of a radiological dispersal device and nuclear sabotage have also been studied (NAS 2015; Purvis 1999; Rosoff and von Winterfeldt 2007; Salter 2001; von Hippel and Schoeppner 2017; Whitehead et al. 2007).

Terrorists might use a variety of means to disperse radiological material (such as from one of the radiological sources used in medicine, industry, or agriculture) over an area. In most cases, there would be few if any radiation-induced deaths from such an event: however, the public fear of radiation means that such an event could have devastatingly disruptive social and economic consequences, potentially amounting to tens of billions of dollars in cleanup and disruption costs. Most of the impact would be the result of public fears of radiation and government reaction, and is therefore difficult to predict with any precision (see Box 4-1). Some analyses suggest that even modest radiation releases would have significant disruptive effects (Giesecke et al. 2012; Trost and Vargas 2020). A risk analysis that includes a characterization of the uncertainties would be helpful in response planning.

BOX 4-1
Impact of Radiological Dispersal Devices: Goiânia, Brazil

A radiological dispersal device can have a strong psychological effect, as demonstrated in an event in Goiânia, Brazil, in which a cesium-137 irradiator (in powder form) was part of a stolen radiotherapy device. The device was stolen for its scrap metal value, and during its dismantlement, the source capsule was ruptured. The scrap metal was sold to a junkyard dealer and, as a consequence, the radioactive powder was widely distributed.

"The authorities set up a radiological screening post in the soccer stadium and announced that anyone concerned about contamination could come in for a free screening. Although the screening was voluntary, and not a public health mandate, 125,800 people in a city of about 1.2 million came forward to be screened. Of those, only 249 were actually contaminated, 20 required hospitalization, and 4 eventually died. The ratio of concerned, anxious, and even panicky people requiring attention to those actually contaminated was approximately 500 to 1. Complicating the picture is the fact that of the first 60,000 who were monitored, 5,000 had psychosomatic reactions, which mimicked symptoms of radiation exposure" (Salter 2001, p. 18).

The effects of a nuclear sabotage event could cover a broad range, from purely economic (as in the insider sabotage that destroyed the turbine at the Doel-4 nuclear plant in Belgium in 2014) to a devastating radiation release comparable to those of the Chernobyl accident. Actions that lead to a fire in a spent fuel pool might be difficult to accomplish, but could be especially devastating. The National Academies of Sciences, Engineering, and Medicine (NASEM 2016) study of the Fukushima disaster focused on security, including security of spent fuel rods, and on the sociological and psychological effects of the accident. Two of its key messages relevant to sabotage and assessing its impacts are reproduced below (NASEM 2016):

> The understanding of security risks at nuclear power plants and spent fuel storage facilities can be improved through risk assessment. Event trees and other representational formalisms can be used to systematically explore terrorist attack scenarios, responses, and potential consequences. Expert elicitation can be used to rank scenarios; develop likelihood estimates; and characterize adaptive adversary responses to various preventive, protective, or deterrence actions. The identification of scenarios may be incomplete, and the estimates developed through expert elicitation are subjective and can have large uncertainties. Nevertheless, risk assessment methods that focus on the risk triplet—scenarios, likelihoods, and consequences—can contribute useful security insights. (Finding 4.1)

> The U.S. nuclear industry and the U.S. Nuclear Regulatory Commission should strengthen their capabilities for identifying, evaluating, and managing the risks from terrorist attacks. Particular attention is needed to broaden scenario identification, including asymmetric attacks; account for the adaptive nature of adversaries; account for the performance of plant security personnel in responding to the identified scenarios; estimate the potential onsite

> and offsite consequences of attack scenarios, including radioactive releases and psychological impacts; and develop strategies for countering the identified threats [emphasis added]. (Recommendation 4.1A)

Analyses of the consequences of nuclear terrorism could also include the effects of a country's actions taken in response to the initial attack. For example, damage of the 9/11 attacks inflicted by al-Qaeda on the United States was not only the loss of life and resources resulting from the direct airplane attacks, but also the subsequent actions by the United States, which led to fighting two prolonged wars with significant economic and human effects, as well as costly homeland security measures.

It is important to note that a concerted terrorist attack could involve several local events with attacks of a different nature, such as the release of radioactive material in one city and a biological attack in another city at the same time.

Damage Effects of Nuclear Weapons

The publicly available nuclear weapons effects analyses funded by the Department of Defense (DoD) between the late 1950s and late 1970s were largely focused on increasing accuracy of damage estimates for U.S. nuclear weapons against adversary targets and the potential effects of an attack on U.S. military forces (Binninger et al. 1974; Murphy et al. 1975). Mathematical models were developed to estimate direct damage and weapons effects that occur immediately or in the hours or days after an explosion. While the weapon effects codes have evolved significantly over time, the codes are still used today: see Binninger et al. (1974) for mathematical model descriptions; Moakler (2015) for descriptions of the evolution of the vulnerability number for thermonuclear kill system; and Helfand et al. (2002) for the consequences assessment tool set system developed by the Federal Emergency Management Agency and the Defense Threat Reduction Agency.

Some observers have noted that additional research is needed to better understand overlooked physical effects. For example, Buddemeier (2010, p. 31) argued:

> Updating our cold war understanding of blast damage in a modern city is another important area of research. The bombings of Hiroshima and Nagasaki demonstrated that the area of glass breakage is nearly 16 times greater than the area of significant structural damage. Injury from broken glass has not previously been well modeled, however, because cold war planners generally considered it not of military significance.

Dresch and Baum (1973) performed a similar analysis with the stated purpose of expanding the damage effects methodologies into analyses of potential economic recovery. Similarly, Eden (2006) documented that the U.S. military primarily emphasized blast effects in assessing the damage from different types of attacks and concluded that DoD systematically understated the impact of fire. For a recent analysis of both the physical and nonphysical consequences of nuclear war, see Scouras et al. (2021).

Weapons Effects Beyond Immediate Damage

Other early consequence analyses expanded the timeline of effects to include those that occur weeks to years after the initial explosions and also expanded the list of effects that were studied. For example, the 1947 U.S. Strategic Bomb Survey's medical effects section included the nature of casualties (e.g., radiation and fires/burns), environmental sanitation (e.g., water supply; sewage and waste disposal such as public sewerage, night soil collection and disposal, and garbage and refuse collection and disposal; milk and food sanitation; insect and rodent control; disposal of the dead; and evacuation), food supply and nutrition, effects on the medical system, communicable diseases, and psychological effects (U.S. Strategic Bombing Surveys 1947). Another early book on the subject expanded this list by assessing the social impact of nuclear bombings, including large-scale nuclear war and the ability for a society to reform and function (Iklé 1958); the book borrows heavily on the U.S. Strategic Bombing Survey.

Significant consequence analyses were conducted in the 1970s and 1980s. The Office of Technology Assessment (OTA 1979) examined the effects of nuclear war on the populations and economies of the United States and the Soviet Union and reached several major conclusions:

- The effects of a nuclear war that cannot be calculated are at least as important as those for which calculations are attempted.
- The impact of even a small or limited nuclear attack, particularly on cities, would be enormous.
- The situation in which the survivors of a nuclear attack find themselves will be unprecedented.
- From an economic point of view, and possibly from a political and social viewpoint as well, conditions after an attack would get worse before they started to get better. This postwar damage could be as devastating as the damage from the actual nuclear explosions.

A compendium of lectures, *The Medical Implications of Nuclear War* (IOM 1986), includes articles on genetic, psychological, social, and economic effects. These early studies show that some researchers (and funders) recognized the importance of and were beginning to explore the social and psychological effects of nuclear war. It is noteworthy and disturbing that there has been so little attention to further deepening understanding of these vital impacts since 1986.

Weapons Effects: Post–Cold War Studies and New Methods

Serious government and academic studies of nuclear weapons consequences all but ceased after the Cold War (Frankel et al. 2015). The terrorist attacks of 9/11 spurred new studies on nuclear terrorism effects, and the "humanitarian consequences of nuclear weapons" movement in the 2000s and 2010s focused renewed attention on the potential effects of nuclear war through a series of international conferences. This led to new examinations of some of these potential effects from scholars all over the world (e.g., Løvold et al. 2013). There was also renewed interest in using quantitative methods for analyzing risks of catastrophic events (Garrick 2008).

Long-Term Effects and Social Phenomena

Some studies show that the long-term and societal consequences of either nuclear war or nuclear or radiological terrorism can far outweigh the immediate and near-term effects in terms of economic and psychological impact. However, the present understanding of these indirect consequences and the ability to model and estimate them remains limited. Furthermore, challenging problems of assessing general societal or psychological consequences have not been identified as a high priority for researchers or funding agencies (Frankel et al. 2015).

Methods for assessing societal and psychological effects have relied on limited data and mostly on the analysis of human behavior in response to other kinds of events. New large-scale computing approaches are beginning to integrate human decision making with infrastructure following an event, and this work offers new insights.

Estimating and calculating the effects of small- and midscale events can be informed by past events, such as Chernobyl, Hiroshima and Nagasaki, or the 9/11 terrorist attacks. However, there are no past events to inform estimates of the consequences of a large-scale nuclear conflict. In short, the ability to comprehend and estimate the magnitude of the effects in the future and to determine their value using analysis is limited, and some argue impossible (Slovic and Lin 2020). Fictional interpretations and human imagination have proven useful media for comprehending, if not predicting, the magnitude of the impact of a large-scale nuclear conflict.[4] This narrative and artistic approach is accessible to a wide audience and conveys emotional content not readily captured by analytical methods.

Estimates of the consequences of nuclear explosions have relied first and foremost on engineering-type methods. Weapons were tested, effects measured, and

[4] Ronald Reagan's reaction that the film *The Day After* both depressed him and affirmed his belief in the importance of a strong deterrent to prevent nuclear war is just one example (Frankel et al. 2015).

calculations done of the impact of such effects on various kinds of structures, on people, and on other items of interest. Nuclear weapons effects analyses funded by DoD between the late 1950s and late 1970s (which are publicly available) were focused on the development of increasingly accurate damage estimates for U.S. nuclear weapons against adversary targets and potential effects on U.S. military forces (Binninger et al. 1974; Dolan 1972; Glasstone and Dolan 1977; Murphy et al. 1975; P.L. 81-920). The effects studied were mainly the direct effects that occur immediately or in the hours or days after an explosion (Frankel et al. 2015).

Mathematical models were developed and refined as better data or more powerful computers became available. However, the more substantive consequences of these weapon effects have not been deeply or extensively explored, if for no other reason than the lack of empirical evidence that can be brought to bear on this problem.

Methods for assessing societal and psychological impacts have relied on surrogate data, including analyzing human behavior in response to other kinds of events. These effects might be heavily dependent on the societies that are affected, their government, and their general attitude and response to catastrophes. New large-scale computing approaches are beginning to offer new insights by better integrating human decision making into analyses of possible events. However, all approaches are limited by the lack of historical data and the corresponding uncertainties (Quinlan 2009).

Prominent among these studies are environmental impact analyses using current climate models, which suggest that in cases in which tens to hundreds of cities are attacked with nuclear weapons, the smoke from burning cities would rise into the upper atmosphere and block a portion of sunlight, altering the global climate for a period of years. The impact on land and in oceans would likely affect agriculture and other food resources, potentially putting hundreds of millions of people at risk of starvation.

This scenario is reminiscent of a nuclear winter, first described in the 1980s; the conclusion of the more recent studies has been to reinforce the earlier findings that were based on far less advanced computer simulations. Indeed, the underlying process of self-lofting of soot proposed by Crutzen and Birks (2016) has now been documented through observations above wildfires: large fires release soot into the lower atmosphere (troposphere), where it absorbs sunlight and becomes warm, thereby warming the surrounding air that then rises, pulling the soot into the upper atmosphere (stratosphere) where it can remain for weeks or months.

Many details about the consequences of nuclear explosion–produced soot remain uncertain, but a key point is that, to this committee's knowledge, this topic has not been extensively studied by the U.S. government, especially regarding the impact on highly interconnected, technologically dependent modern society, as well as on climate.[5]

A study of the social, economic, and health impacts of a 10-kiloton improvised nuclear device was undertaken as a part of a U.S. National Planning Scenario. Individual and collective behaviors were modeled and their interactions with the built infrastructure were investigated from up to 48 hours to roughly 1 week after the event.[6] Agent-based models, social network analysis, and machine learning technologies were developed to build digital twins of functioning city-scale systems. Individuals' behaviors were represented as a partially observable Markov decision process, in which the evolution of a system from one state to another is assumed to depend only on the first, and the system state at any time is uncertain. The model allows for an analysis of the effects of future decisions. Collective behavior is represented by connecting these individual models using an underlying network. Each individual is part of multiple networks. Conceptually, a person has a social network and associated behavioral representation corresponding to an infrastructure. For example, individual behavior related to a communication network would represent whom a person might call, how often, ownership of a cell phone, and other characteristics of human-communication interactions.

These systems are data driven, and the models are informed by available numerical and procedural data. Analytical techniques are then developed to derive insights from these agent-based simulations. Ideas from statistical designs are used to create a set of computational experiments and the outcomes of the analysis scenarios are computed, not just as point estimates but as trajectories and collective behavioral outcomes, along with the corresponding uncertainties. For example, one may be interested in how a family is reconstituted, or the number of injured individuals who seek medical care at a given triage center.

Psychological and Social Effects

Yet another type of study involves the psychological effects of nuclear events: for example, Becker (2012) reviews and reexamines earlier social and psychological studies with new analogies and updated analyses. The social and psychological effects of large-scale nuclear weapons events continue to be difficult to assess (e.g., Slovic and Lin 2020). The methods used for psychological and social impact studies

[5] This committee did not further consider climate impact in its work because the National Defense Authorization Act for Fiscal Year 2021 called for the National Academies to conduct a separate, detailed study of the nonfallout atmospheric effects of scenarios for nuclear war, ranging from low-quantity regional exchanges to large-scale exchanges between major powers.

[6] The outcome of these initial studies will play a role in developing future models that range from weeks to years.

largely extrapolate behaviors from other radiation emergencies (e.g., nuclear accidents) and from other relevant situations (e.g., releases of invisible toxic agents, etc.). In addition, the work takes into account the literature on the mental health effects of Hiroshima and Nagasaki. The studies of these effects are essential since there were many lessons learned from the immediate and long-term effects of the nuclear bombing and the recovery paths of both cities. Nuclear events are closely tied to stress, anxiety, depression, and other mental and emotional health outcomes, all of which can lead to other health complications (Lambiase et al. 2014).

Areas of social and psychological research have expanded to help explore such questions as the ability and willingness of responders to be involved in radiological and nuclear incidents, or how to provide effective messaging and communication to the general public and responders following a nuclear event. This work uses a variety of methods, from focus groups, interviews, and surveys to analysis of how text messages are received and processed.[7] However, the long-term and psychological, societal, and political consequences of nuclear weapons use are not well understood.

THE CHALLENGES OF ASSESSING THE OVERALL RISKS OF NUCLEAR WAR AND NUCLEAR TERRORISM

Factors of Complexity in Risk Analysis

The consequences of nuclear weapons use are qualitatively different from those of any other form of conflict. Therefore, the risks of triggering nuclear weapons use and the conditions under which it might arise are also profoundly different from those of nonnuclear (i.e., conventional) war or terrorism.

This section aims *not* to address the causes and associated risks of war or terrorism in general, but to focus on those that might lead to nuclear detonations or dispersal. All evaluations of potential causes and risks are necessarily speculative. It is possible and perhaps even likely that a future nuclear conflict may erupt for reasons completely overlooked by current analyses. Nevertheless, the implications of nuclear weapons use are so enormous that they deserve thorough attention, ranging from technical and military analysis to legal, social, political, environmental, and ethical considerations.

[7] For collections of information on nuclear and radiological response, see the TRACIE Healthcare Emergency Preparedness Information Gateway, hosted by the Department of Health and Human Services at https://asprtracie.hhs.gov.

Coevolution of Risk Assessment and Actions

Assessing the risks of a nuclear war or a nuclear terrorism event is fundamentally different from assessing the risks of natural events, such as an earthquake or tornado, because decisions, policies, and actions of individual and collective human agents affect the risks more directly. The assessment for natural events is challenging because of uncertainties in understanding the physical processes, but complex computational models (complete with the assessment of uncertainties) have been in use for more than 50 years (Cornell 1968; McGuire 2008). There are some analytical lessons to be learned about the effect of large disasters from the assessment of seismic risks. In the case of earthquakes, society can affect the outcome to the degree that it understands the seismic loads and the uncertainties involved by enforcing building codes, which can increase the capacity of the different structures to absorb these loads, to some extent. This is true, in particular, for the seismic reinforcement of nuclear power plants, which is supported in each case by a site-specific risk analysis. The effects of social and political actions in preparation for and response to natural catastrophes can be observed across different countries. However, the social and political actions involved in nuclear war and nuclear terrorism and the scale, as well as the coevolution of realities and risk perceptions in such complex systems, makes assessing the risks especially challenging.

Moreover, there are significant disagreements among experts regarding the effects of relatively fundamental nuclear force decisions on nuclear security. For example, does procuring more nuclear weapons or developing ballistic missile defenses increase or decrease risks? These policy choices are interdependent, coevolving, and difficult to assess.

Cross-Domain Interactions and the Impact of Modern Technologies

The unique characteristics of nuclear weapons may have complex interactions with emerging or disruptive technologies, which can affect the initiation of war, the perceived value or necessity of preemption, incentives for nuclear weapons use, the restoration of deterrence, and conflict termination (Roberts 2021).

Types of threats can be intertwined, such as some nations having threatened nuclear retaliation in order to deter attacks with biological or chemical, as well as nuclear, weapons. Cyber and space infrastructures are closely and increasingly connected, and an attack on one domain can compromise the other. For example, a nuclear crisis could involve a cyber attack, such as an attack on space capabilities associated with nuclear surveillance and warning; an attack on command, control, and communications; an intrusion into cyber systems for purposes of intelligence gathering; or intrusions into conventional capabilities that may also threaten nuclear command and communications systems. In these and other instances, a cyber attack could be misunderstood or misattributed, especially if it takes place during a period of otherwise increased tension between nuclear adversaries.

One way of trying to deter threats to the U.S. nuclear infrastructure is to protect critical military or civilian infrastructure. A nuclear, conventional, or cyber attack on such infrastructure could be considered serious enough to trigger nuclear retaliation, because the published postures of both the United States and Russia could be taken to imply this possibility. Yet what constitutes critical infrastructure and what conditions would justify a nuclear response remain unspecified.

To some observers, ambiguity in posture is a benefit for deterrence, because avoiding specificity about the actions that would trigger nuclear response is viewed as complicating prospective adversaries' planning of an attack. To others, such ambiguity is an invitation for misunderstanding and misinterpretation, especially at times of tension, let alone crisis between nuclear powers, and all the more so in the presence of accidents or human error.

New technologies have vastly improved sensing, monitoring, communications, and warning—all of which can reduce risks of crisis or conflict. However, these technologies may offer new paths to crisis and, potentially, to conflict and therefore the possibility of nuclear weapons use. The rapidly increasing diversity of new technologies in space, cyber, and other domains provides new pathways to instability and crisis, through the increased power and reach of these technologies, their interconnectedness and widespread commercial usage, and their increased accessibility to nations around the world. One of the key uncertainties when assessing the nuclear risks over the next 10 years is anticipating emerging and developing technologies and their impacts.

Likely Pathways to Nuclear War

Many dangerous pathways could lead to the use of nuclear weapons. Exploring these scenarios is part of developing risk analysis methods, and the list of examples described here is neither complete nor definitive. Analysts have to address how evolving technologies and changing geopolitics are changing those dangers, and what steps could be taken to reduce the risks that such technologies pose. Each nation develops its own assessment of those risks, as well as its own assessment of what its adversaries' potential actions might be.

Some pathways may involve escalation from a crisis to a conventional military conflict, and from that conflict to nuclear weapons use. Events of recent years seem to make clear that future serious crises and conflicts will probably be complex, multidomain events, and they are likely to feature cyber attacks and disinformation campaigns starting in "the gray zone," as well as more traditional military operations (Gerasimov 2016). In addition, multiple parties may be involved, including allies of the contending nuclear states or other states or terrorist groups seeking to take advantage of the situation.

The following are characteristics of technologies that could increase the risk that nuclear war would occur:

- *Technologies that make deterrent forces vulnerable or that create an incentive to strike first in a particular domain*: Threats of both cyber and counterspace technologies can add to the risks of crisis escalation.
- *Technologies that blur the lines between peace and conflict, or between different levels of conflict*: Cyber activities, in particular, are blurring conflict lines as the United States and its adversaries are in each other's information systems every day, even in peacetime. It is unclear what kinds of attacks would represent an escalation. In some cases, cyber assaults can (perhaps inadvertently) damage computer systems, which might be seen as an escalation requiring a serious response.
- *Technologies that entangle conventional and nuclear forces and command and control*: With dual-use weapons and command systems, attacks seen by one side as essential to preventing a conventional conflict can be seen by the other side as threatening its nuclear capabilities. Even worse, such attacks could be seen as part of a large-scale attack that might require a nuclear response.
- *Technologies that compress the time for decision or worsen the decision environment*: In some circumstances, decisions in a potentially nuclear crisis will have to be made quickly. Future systems enabled by artificial intelligence may help the decision maker respond quickly but could also introduce biases and flawed information (e.g., "hallucinations") into decision making.
- *Technologies that proliferate nuclear weapons*: If there are more nations, groups, or individuals that can decide to use nuclear weapons, the routes to nuclear conflict increase rapidly in number, diversity, and complexity. The global effort to stem the spread of nuclear weapons—including keeping them out of terrorists' hands— continues to be justified despite having been remarkably successful to date.

Finally, when a nation's decision makers think about what forces to build and what operations to undertake, they are often thinking mainly about strengthening the deterrence threat that their nation poses to its adversaries and the capability that it offers to reassure its allies. But one must remember the security dilemma: what looks like a defensive step to strengthen one nation's deterrent might look like an offensive threat to its adversaries, potentially provoking them to respond. Part of China's motivation for its current nuclear buildup, for example, appears to be intended to counter the threat to its forces from U.S. counterforce capabilities and missile defenses.

Traditional arms control is problematic for some of these evolving technologies. For example, one cannot count, measure, or control capabilities in the cyber domain. As a consequence, most risk reduction is likely to come from unilateral steps—each nation making sure that its own forces are secure and resilient against cyber and counterspace systems.

However, there may be room for rules of the road or confidence-building measures that reduce the risks posed by emerging technologies. Bilateral and multilateral talks on cyber security are ongoing, as part of a broader umbrella of strategic stability conversations. Unilateral steps can also play a crucial role in enhancing strategic stability, starting with building mutual confidence, especially during periods of animosity between rival nations.[8] Still, future rounds of nuclear arms control may require at least *some* clearer understanding on how to control nonnuclear technologies that affect nuclear dangers—including hypersonic weapon systems, missile defenses, long-range precision conventional weapons, counterspace systems, and cyber capabilities.

Wargaming and simulations continue to have a role in improving each nation's understanding of how these emerging technologies—applied in different geostrategic contexts—might contribute to risks of conflict and of escalation. While the complex factors involved in decision making are difficult to represent fully, these and other approaches may provide benefits from evolving technologies while moderating to some degree the risks they may cause.

Challenges in Assessing the Risks of Nuclear Terrorism

A wide range of challenges confront assessments of the probability of nuclear terrorism. There are strong disagreements even on the direction of the trend: some analysts argue that major improvements in security for nuclear weapons and materials and the killing or capture of the top of leadership of al-Qaeda and the Islamic State have greatly reduced the probability of nuclear terrorism, while others argue that factors decreasing the chances are more than balanced by factors increasing them.

The potential consequences from nuclear or radiological terrorism would cover a broad spectrum, from minor to catastrophic. While the direct consequences of physical effects of nuclear explosives are reasonably well understood, the long-term

[8] An example in the space domain is the April 18, 2022, U.S. announcement that it unilaterally "commits not to conduct destructive, direct-ascent anti-satellite (ASAT) missile testing" (White House 2022).

economic, environmental, political, and social consequences are perhaps more devastating and are poorly understood.

The challenges in assessing the risks of nuclear terrorism described below focus primarily on a terrorist detonation of a nuclear bomb, but similar challenges would face efforts to assess the risks of other forms of nuclear or radiological terrorism.

Uncertain Terrorist Capabilities and Motivations

As discussed above, past terrorist groups have pursued nuclear weapons and radiological dispersal devices and plotted to sabotage nuclear facilities. Nevertheless, most of those reported events are now decades in the past. Assessing current and future intentions is challenging because terrorist activities take place in secret and groups can change rapidly.

Uncertain Availability of Nuclear Weapons or Materials

In the 1990s, there were multiple seizures of kilogram quantities of stolen plutonium or highly enriched uranium, nearly all of which appear to have come from the former Soviet Union. It has been a decade since the last well-documented seizure of stolen highly enriched uranium, amounting to a few tens of grams (in Moldova in 2011). Does that mean that terrorists could no longer get weapons-usable nuclear materials? Or, as some suspect, is enough material for a bomb still outside state control, at unknown locations?

With ongoing incidents around the world in which terrorists manage to overcome security at very well-guarded nonnuclear sites, what are the odds that the same might happen at a nuclear site in the future? There have been significant advances in approaches to modeling and testing the effectiveness of nuclear security and accounting systems in recent decades, but the latest approaches are still applied unevenly around the world. And thieves at nonnuclear facilities often succeed in defeating security systems using unforeseen tactics. Modeling and assessment are better able to assess the effectiveness of security at one site relative to another than they are able to assess the absolute probability of a successful theft or sabotage at any particular location. Even judgments on relative effectiveness are uncertain, however, for at least three reasons: (1) the vulnerabilities that adversaries end up exploiting may be ones those doing security assessments have not thought of; (2) one site may have better protection against one type of threat and another better protection against a different type, and which approaches are most likely is not well understood; and (3) often, day-to-day security performance is different from performance when an inspection or assessment is being carried out.

Methods for assessing how likely it is that, after a theft, adversaries would be able to successfully get nuclear material or components to a terrorist group wanting to make a bomb are much less mature. How would sellers with nuclear material and potential buyers find each other? How would they have confidence that the other party was not a government agent participating in a sting operation? What are the chances that nuclear material would be detected and recovered, and how do those chances vary from one part of the world to another? There are few data for answering these questions or for judging whether the stolen nuclear material that has been intercepted represents close to 100 percent or only a small fraction of the total material stolen over time. Various analogies (such as drug smuggling) have been used to try to make judgments on this point, but the situations are often quite different.

Uncertain Difficulty of Making, Delivering, and Detonating a Nuclear Bomb

Similarly, there is broad disagreement over how likely it is that, once a terrorist group had obtained nuclear material, they would be able to turn it into at least a crude nuclear bomb; how likely it is that they would be able to deliver that weapon to a target site in the face of efforts to stop them; how likely it is that they would choose to actually detonate such a weapon rather than keeping it for deterrence and blackmail; and how likely it is that the bomb would actually go off. Data for assessing these probabilities are simply not available.

Uncertain Economic, Political, Environmental, and Social Consequences

The consequences of acts of nuclear and radiological terrorism are difficult to fully grasp. In the case of an actual nuclear detonation, a good deal is known about the direct effects that would result. But, as discussed elsewhere in this report, the reverberating economic, political, and social consequences, not only in the country attacked but elsewhere around the world, are difficult to understand and predict. As just one of many possible consequences, after a nuclear detonation, once people understand that the nuclear material for the bomb would fit in a briefcase, traditional notions of civil liberties and protection from unreasonable search and seizure may be swept aside by demands for enhanced security.

There have been important efforts to model the potential impacts of an attack with a radiological dispersal device or a release from an accident or sabotage at a major nuclear facility. In the case of releases from nuclear facilities, there is real-world experience from the Chernobyl and Fukushima disasters to draw on. But understanding of the full scope of the impact on society of such events—particularly if they were malevolent rather than accidental, and people feared further attacks would occur—is still in its early stages. The conceptual framework known as *the social amplification of risk* may provide useful guidance for improved modeling (Kasperson et al. 1988; Pidgeon et al. 2003).

Interacting Uncertainties

As with nuclear war, all the uncertainties about the risks of nuclear terrorism may interact with each other. If, for example, adversaries believe that nuclear weapons and weapons-usable nuclear material would be very hard to get, they are likely to put less effort into recruiting the people who might be able to help figure out how to detonate a stolen nuclear weapon or put together a crude nuclear bomb. If defenders are underestimating the potential consequences of nuclear terrorism, they are likely to require fewer measures to protect against it, which may increase its probability.

Lack of Direct Evidence

As described in Chapter 2, the evidence needed to support risk analyses can be drawn from many sources: statistical evidence, past near misses and false alerts, surrogate data, models, war games, red teaming, and expert judgment. In the case of nuclear war and nuclear terrorism, however, direct evidence is limited. Some past near misses and false alerts may involve factors that are still relevant, thus providing some statistical information, but expert judgment and assumptions are likely to be needed to bridge the inevitable gaps in the evidence available. For assessments of the overall risks of nuclear war and nuclear terrorism, uncertainties in the available evidence can be large, and experience in other fields may offer an important part of that evidence.

Uncertainties about the assumptions and inputs to a risk model can be represented in the risk analysis. The lack of direct evidence may make it difficult or impossible to accurately consider important dependencies across relevant scenarios, but the existence of these dependencies needs to be highlighted when presenting the results to decision makers.

CONCLUSIONS

CONCLUSION 4-1: There is a need to improve the understanding of less-well-understood physical effects of nuclear weapons (such as fires; damage in modern urban environments; electromagnetic pulse effects; and climatic effects, such as nuclear winter), as well as the assessment and estimation of psychological, societal, and political consequences of nuclear weapons use.

CONCLUSION 4-2: The U.S. government and the international community have invested significant resources and time in trying to understand and reduce the risks of nuclear war and nuclear terrorism. The risks remain real and are becoming more complex as new technologies and new adversaries arise.

CONCLUSION 4-3: There is a fundamental lack of direct evidence about nuclear war and nuclear terrorism. Analysts attempt to mitigate the resulting uncertainties by applying different methods and using multiple sources of information to supplement the limited body of evidence.

Given this lack of evidence, an analysis of overall risks of nuclear war or nuclear terrorism is likely to involve great uncertainties about the likelihood and the range of consequences of relevant scenarios. As discussed above, some physical consequences of nuclear weapons use are well understood, but significant uncertainties remain, especially regarding the psychological, societal, environmental, and political consequences of nuclear weapons use.

All risk analyses involve uncertainty, and communicating those uncertainties is essential. The specific quantitative result of an analysis of the overall risks of nuclear war or nuclear terrorism may have little or no policy relevance. If decision makers are reluctant or unable to consider the significant uncertainties and effects involved in such an analysis, the utility of such an overall estimate is unclear. Still, structuring the risk problem, exploring the possible scenarios, and identifying what gaps in evidence are addressable may be of great value to decision makers to prioritize risk mitigation actions.

CONCLUSION 4-4: Assessing the overall risks of nuclear war and nuclear terrorism involves great uncertainties about the likelihood and consequences of different scenarios. The assessment and communications of these uncertainties are critical for policy decisions essential to managing these risks.

Although overall analyses of the risks of nuclear war or nuclear terrorism may have limited policy relevance, analyses of specific risk problems related to nuclear war and nuclear terrorism are routinely requested and used by the U.S. government. As noted in Chapter 2, the framing and formulation of a risk problem is a critical first step in risk analysis. Well-formulated risk problems addressing specific questions can allow analysts to overcome the challenges posed by the lack of direct evidence. Chapter 6 addresses these specific risk questions and the methods analysts may use to address them.

CONCLUSION 4-5: The value of risk analysis is not solely in assessing the overall risks of nuclear war or nuclear terrorism. Risk analysis can also provide valuable input on many specific problems related to nuclear war and nuclear terrorism, including an understanding of the uncertainties involved.

5

The Structure of Risk Analysis

In this chapter, the committee reviews the basic components of risk analysis, including definitions, how risk analyses are structured, the main sources of evidence for risk analyses related to nuclear war or terrorism, and the assumptions involved in risk analysis.

RISK DEFINITIONS

Risk is a complex and often controversial concept, derived from the existence of a hazard, and its fundamental characteristic is the uncertainty of possible undesirable events and their outcomes. Risk analysis generally includes a description of the possible events and hazards with the associated probabilities and consequences of such events. "Risk" is used to represent a set of related, but distinct ideas. When using the term, speakers and risk analysts may be referring to a number of meanings (DHS 2017) and focus on different aspects of the term, including

- *Hazards*: risk as the result of a hazard or set of hazards. For example, "How should we rank the risks that we all face when we need to set priorities?"
- *Event likelihood*: the likelihood of an unfortunate occurrence. For example, "What is the risk of nuclear explosion in our lifetime?"
- *Event outcome*: risk as a consequence. For example, "What are the risks—especially, the consequences—of the detonation of an improvised nuclear device in a densely populated city center?"

- *Both the likelihood and the possible outcomes*: risk as a function of both the likelihood and the severity of the consequences of an activity. For example, "How great is the risk of damage to a house in an earthquake, taking into account both the severity of damage that might occur and its likelihood?"

The committee uses the term "risk"—following Kaplan and Garrick (1981) with the addition of the time horizon in which these events might happen following Paté-Cornell (2011)—to refer to four questions:

1. What can happen? Specifically, what can go wrong? This is the scenario identification or description.
2. How likely is it that these events will happen? This is the probability of that scenario.
3. If these events happen, what are the potential consequences? This is the consequence or evaluation measure of that scenario.
4. What is the time horizon in which these events might happen?

In the realm of nuclear and radiological weapons, the hazard is the existence of nuclear material, design, engineering, production, and equipment that allows for the real or threatened manufacturing and launching of nuclear weapons, as well as the use or threatened use of a nuclear or radiological device for terrorist attacks.

The level of severity for a nuclear war or terrorist incident depends on the kind and number of weapon(s) that are used, the nature and number of target(s) affected, and the immediate and long-term consequences (physical, social, psychological, economic, political, cultural, and environmental). The level of severity can vary significantly—for instance, from the use of a single small-scale nuclear weapon to incapacitate an enemy on the battlefield to the nuclear destruction of several big cities by strategic weapons.

In some cases, risk may be described solely by the probability of an event in a given time period (e.g., in a given year, how likely is a nuclear terrorist attack?), or by a quantitative description of both the probability and consequences of the event (Paté-Cornell 1996). Such a quantitative description of a risk can be a complementary cumulative probability distribution, continuous or discrete, which represents the probability that different levels of consequences are exceeded in a given time unit or time horizon.

RISK ANALYSIS AS A SYSTEMATIC PROCESS

Risk analysis is a systematic process designed to comprehend the risk mechanisms associated with a hazard or threat and to express that risk, based on available evidence and knowledge, to inform decision making. Risk analysis is used across many domains and relies on a logical, systematic accounting of event dependencies and the dynamics of different possible scenarios. The power of a risk analysis is in providing a systematic framework for making clear the assumptions and evidence (imperfect as it may be) used to identify and assess the risks. Done well, risk analyses separate the risk characterization from the value judgments made by decision makers and stakeholders. Risk analyses do not dictate decisions; they inform them.

Risk analysis requires structuring a risk problem and systematically considering a number of interdependent or independent factors and scenarios. The objective is to clarify the assumptions and their effects on the results and to identify information that needs to be gathered (in the time available) to improve the understanding of the uncertainties involved.

A vital part of risk assessment is framing—formulation of the structure of the problem, the dependencies among the elements, and the possible external factors all must be considered. Risk assessment and management standards are available (ASIS 2015; ISO 2018). A successful assessment might also uncover important gaps that need to be addressed by gathering new evidence or a previously unrecognized interplay of components of the problem. An appropriately structured risk analysis brings transparency to the assumptions, scenarios, data, methods, and results. It permits verifying the sources of information for different parts of the problem and understanding the different models that were developed, the effect of the assumptions, and the effects of external events and circumstances.

The work of a risk analysis team is thus to identify the key components of the question being posed, formulate the analytical models, and characterize uncertainties as best as they can—including recognition of the limits of the analysis. Relevant statistical data may exist for some parts of the problem, but other inputs and sources of information, including surrogate data, models, and expert judgment, may be needed, especially for complex problems.

The results of a risk assessment can be either quantitative or qualitative. For example, when analyzing probabilities, qualitative results are described by words (such as "frequently," "unlikely," "low," or "high"). Quantitative results can represent different types of results, such as the probability of exceeding different levels of damage per time unit.

Risk analysis supports decision making through a systematic decomposition of the problem into scenarios and assessing the risk variations associated with different options. This is done by identifying a set of scenarios that attempt to span the scope of the risk events to be considered in the analysis. Analysts then characterize the uncertainties and consequences of hazardous events, relying on a variety of techniques. In particular, risk analyses may allow identifying risk reduction measures and their effectiveness, computed as a difference of risk results with and without the considered options. Done well, the values and assumptions underlying a risk characterization are transparent, and the risk analyses can help separate the risk characterization from the value judgments made by decision makers and stakeholders.

Of course, a risk analysis can be poorly done and lead to questionable results. It is critical that the results not be inadvertently biased by the analysts, such as truncating databases to eliminate inconvenient possibilities (see National Research Council 1996; Slovic 1990).

Risk analysis is a relatively new tool in human history. Humans have always had to navigate a dangerous world. Acquired knowledge and intuitive understanding of risks (combined with fear and other emotions) served as a compass to guide protective actions. There was—and still is—no time to ponder when one hears an ominous sound in a bush or heavy footsteps in the night. Over time, humans have developed a more analytic approach to these concepts, including probability and risk, which could bring science and analytic thinking (time permitting) to supplement experience, intuition, and emotion.

In the 18th century, Reverend Thomas Bayes applied laws of logic to show how a conditional probability (e.g., the probability of an event A given a signal B) could be simply expressed as the ratio of the joint probability of A and B divided by the probability of B. That simple formula and its derivations allow the computation of the probability of a scenario composed of several events, accounting for possible interdependencies.

Some early applications of Bayesian methods were developed in the 1940s by the British intelligence services to break the Japanese and German codes and develop strategic and tactical protections of maritime convoys across the Atlantic. Bayesian probability was formally defined by Savage (1954) and de Finetti (1974). The methods were developed further, including in the form of game analysis in response to the arms race with the Soviet Union that followed World War II.

One of the first systematic risk analyses of an engineered system was developed to support the choices of designers and engineers striving to improve the safety of nuclear power plants (NRC 1975). This study stimulated the further development and application of what became known as probabilistic risk assessment (NRC 1975).

Later, in the space industry, these methods were used to minimize the risk of space flights by assessing the risk of failure of rockets and spacecraft, and assigning probabilities to catastrophic consequences. These risk analyses were applied, for instance, to the U.S. Space Shuttle and the International Space Station. However, the results were not always implemented—for instance, recommendations made in an existing risk analysis could have mitigated the risk of the Columbia shuttle accident (Paté-Cornell and Fischbeck 1994).

AVAILABLE SOURCES OF EVIDENCE

Evidence to support risk analyses for nuclear war and nuclear terrorism may be drawn from many sources, but direct evidence in war situations is—thankfully—limited to the nuclear bombing of Hiroshima and Nagasaki. Given the time since those events and the changes in the world, this limited evidence base leaves great uncertainty in assessments of the current risks of nuclear war and nuclear terrorism. Risk analyses include, whenever possible, statistical data relevant to scenarios. They also rely on past experience and near misses (focusing on the parts of these scenarios that are still relevant today), on surrogate data, models, exercises, and expert opinion: all of these can serve as input to a formal risk analysis of systems and policies, including estimates of the consequences of possible scenarios. In the case of nuclear war and nuclear terrorism, large uncertainties remain.

Statistical Evidence

Statistical data, if they exist and are both relevant and sufficient, are of great value to risk analysis. For many scientific and technical questions, there are some statistical data that are relevant to understanding risks relating to nuclear war and terrorism. For example, there is information that helps characterize the materials used in weapons or the effectiveness of border portals that detect smuggled nuclear material.

The validity of statistical data, however, assumes that the system has not changed—as a result of changing policies and technologies, discovered deficiencies in the system, or geopolitical circumstances, for a few examples. It also requires that enough information exists about past events to extract what is still relevant today. While it cannot generally be assumed that the systems are unchanged, past events and near misses can still provide relevant information.

For example, data from previous nuclear tests and the radiation emitted from them can be relevant in understanding current nuclear systems, even if the overall systems are different today. Similarly, past nuclear incidents that did not lead to a conflict can provide information on processes and human reactions that can inform policies and systems under new circumstances. It is important, however, to consider such past near misses as statistical data only after scrutiny to ensure that they are applicable to the new circumstances.

Statistical evidence can be thought of as the result of a statistical analysis using appropriate observations or measurements. The quality and appropriateness of the statistical analysis need to be considered, as well as the quality and appropriateness of the data.

Conventions for communicating risks can also pose a complication, particularly when academic decision analysts work with national security professionals (Friedman et al. 2017).

Past Near Misses and False Alerts

Past near misses and false alerts may inform estimates of the likelihood of future events pertaining to nuclear war and nuclear terrorism, in part because they might point to some potential weaknesses that still exist. Yet, as the circumstances may have changed in response to past events, there may be a wide range of interpretations of these past events. Causes of past failures may have been remedied—by improvement of technical communications, for example—and yet egregious oversights, biases, or flawed assumptions may remain as unrecognized sources of systematic error. Similarly, the systems and practices that other nations have developed and implemented following such near misses or false alerts may have changed or may still be evolving.

Moreover, evidence related to past near misses and false alerts may not be readily available or complete. For example, the Global Terrorism Database of the University of Maryland lists 13 events involving radiological weapons[1]: 10 involved one individual who, over a 3-day period, sent envelopes containing radioactive minerals to government offices in Japan in an attempt to draw attention to alleged smuggling of nuclear materials to North Korea; the other 3 occurred over more than a decade's period in the United States and Europe. The information available in this database is evidently sparse and heterogeneous. The International Atomic Energy Agency also maintains an Incident and Trafficking Database,[2] but this database relies on voluntary reporting by its member states, and it is both incomplete and not limited to terrorism. For example, it includes incidents involving illegal transportation of radioactive material across national borders, and loss or discovery of radioactive materials that should have been under safeguards.

While the interpretation of historical episodes may help analysts identify potential weaknesses or vulnerabilities, these interpretations are subject to the judgment of risk analysts and rely on available (often limited) information.

Surrogate Data

Surrogate data can potentially be used to estimate the corresponding phenomena in the scenarios considered, as long as the differences between the scenarios

[1] See the Global Terrorism Database website at https://www.start.umd.edu/gtd.

[2] See International Atomic Energy Agency, "Incident and Trafficking Database (ITDB)," https://www.iaea.org/resources/databases/itdb.

are taken into account. As an example, while the delivery systems used for nuclear weapons are not tested with nuclear payloads, their reliability and performance can be characterized by looking at tests with inert payloads while accounting for the known differences.

Models

Models are used to represent many important aspects of scenarios as well as systems, so the choice of models is critical for risk analyses. For analyses related to nuclear war or nuclear terrorism, models might represent engineered systems, cyber attacks based on vulnerabilities given a system's structure, conflict development, human behaviors, environmental factors, radiation dispersions, or many other important aspects of the analysis. The models chosen need to include interdependencies among events and external factors that affect the probabilities and consequences of different scenarios.

War Games

Wargaming approaches assume a set of parameters and rules, and allow participants to make decisions and respond to the consequences of those decisions in the context of the game. These are well-studied techniques for exploring the threat landscape and assessing response and mitigation strategies. These tools can help identify possible threats and provide some information about the ease or difficulty of a possible attack and the response to an attack, but do not directly place probabilities on particular scenarios or outcomes.

War games have been used in designing and assessing security systems for nuclear weapons, materials, and facilities. Tabletop exercises and computer simulations are used to assess different possible defense approaches, to identify possible adversary tactics that may be most difficult to defend against, and to train new staff or government officials. While realistic force-on-force exercises are so expensive and disruptive that only a few can be done, tabletop exercises or computer simulations—with individuals playing roles supported by models and simulation to adjudicate player moves—can be conducted for many scenarios.

Wargaming can be especially useful for exploring the conditions in which one party or another in a conflict might decide to use nuclear weapons. A variety of scenarios can be tested with different arrays of nonnuclear and nuclear forces and different strategies on each side. Computer-supported methods make it possible to run large numbers of games and generate results about their outcomes.

Wargaming can thus be undertaken to provide input to a quantitative model from which qualitative information is derived. It is important to note that this approach does not consider the spectrum of all event sequences that can occur in a changing external context. Rather, such methods typically consider a single scenario that results from the choices of the players, but there may be many other branches in these scenarios depending on the choices and ideologies of the players (Emery 2021).

Red Teaming

Red teaming is a method designed to detect vulnerabilities that an adversary can use to achieve its objective. For nuclear war, red teaming means assigning a group to think like the adversaries and to come up with strategies that the adversaries might use to achieve their objectives (Caffrey 2000; Sandoz 2001; Zenko 2015). It is another potentially useful method to structure thinking about some aspects of the risks of a nuclear war, challenge assumptions about plans, and estimate weapon effectiveness. For example, what factors might lead Russia, North Korea, or China to consider the use of nuclear weapons in a conflict with the United States or another country?

For nuclear terrorism, red teaming is used to explore the effectiveness of security systems designed to prevent nuclear or radiological theft or sabotage. It can, for example, provide input regarding the methods adversaries might use to attempt to break into nuclear material storage spaces, or how insiders might attempt to or sabotage a facility. The technique can expose vulnerabilities that might be exploited.

Expert Judgment

Risk analysis for questions related to nuclear war and nuclear terrorism necessarily relies on qualitative and quantitative judgments made by both subject-matter experts and risk analysts. Expert judgment is central to structuring the key components of risk decisions to address such questions as what objectives matter and what choice options should be considered to achieve those objectives. Judgments are then critical to the assessment of the likelihoods of the components of scenarios, their potential consequences, the way these outcomes are described, and the values that are assigned to them.

Analyzing the risks of nuclear war and nuclear terrorism frequently calls for estimates, ranges, or probability distributions for highly uncertain events about which there is no clear consensus or high-quality and sufficient data sources. Examples include estimating the likelihood that a particular nation or group possesses or can acquire weapons of mass destruction, the military strength of state actors, and the capabilities and intent of terrorist groups.

In dealing with analyses based on expert opinion, it is important to understand how the experts were chosen, to what extent they reflect the range of opinions (both technical and political) in the community, and how the expert elicitation was conducted to recognize and guard against biases. The experts should be asked to assess specific factors of the risk scenarios for which they have relevant experience, and decision makers need to be informed of the competence and credibility of the experts.

Challenges to the Elicitation and Use of Expert Opinion

Given the important role that expert opinion often plays in the analysis of risks related to nuclear war and nuclear terrorism (Argyris and French 2017; Downes and Hobbs 2017; Woo 2021), this section highlights some of the conceptual and technical challenges in developing useful and accurate information derived from expert elicitation. The historic approach for dealing with expert opinion and its aggregation is well described in the literature (e.g., Hora 2007; O'Hagan et al. 2006; see also NRC 1990, for an early discussion of the use of these methods in the nuclear power industry).

In integrating expert opinion for use in a risk analysis, some means must be found to summarize the viewpoints across the community (Clemen and Winkler 1999), whether through behavioral strategies for reaching consensus, such as the Delphi method (Rowe and Wright 1999); through mathematical methods of aggregating divergent opinions, such as weighted averaging (Colson and Cooke 2017; Cooke 1991); or a Bayesian combination. The challenges include avoiding undue influence from individuals with forceful personalities (rather than actual expertise) (Wittenbaum and Stasser 1996) and managing the effects of group polarization (Sniezek 1992). In addition, the elicitation method needs to be carefully structured so that the participating experts can accomplish their task (O'Hagan et al. 2006); indeed, many experts are not accustomed to providing their judgment in a quantitative form and may resist doing so (Walker et al. 2001). Classification of nuclear weapons information can also restrict the accuracy and full understanding of the context.

Mellers and colleagues (2014) have shown that, in the long run, quantitative forecasts allow one to measure the relative accuracy of forecasts by different individuals or organizations. Of course, in the nuclear context there have been few actual events, so one can question whether there are enough data for this methodology to be useful. However, insisting on explicit descriptions of possible outcomes and their assessed probabilities and maintaining unclassified aspects of these data in accessible form would allow some long-term analysis of the accuracy of such assessments.

It is widely recognized that expert elicitations, like all individual intuitions, tend to be derived from mental strategies or heuristics that are subject to a variety of serious judgmental biases (Kahneman et al. 1982). There are four known heuristics that lead to biases: availability, representativeness, probability neglect, and framing (Kadane and Wolfson 1998).

Availability

Probability and frequency judgments are biased upward for events that are easier to recall or to imagine happening (Tversky and Kahneman 1973), and even more so when the event is emotionally powerful (Lichtenstein et al. 1978). An inability to recall or imagine important pathways to failure can lead fault trees to underestimate the overall failure probability (Fischhoff et al. 1978).

Representativeness

People may judge the likelihood of an event by the similarity of the image conveyed by the evidence to an idealized or easily imagined image (Tversky and Kahneman 1974). For example, a woman described as interested in social justice may well be judged more likely to be a bank teller and a feminist than to be either a bank teller or a feminist. This is logically impossible, as the conjunction of two events cannot be more probable than either event alone. As a scenario becomes more detailed, it tends to be seen as more coherent and realistic, and thus more probable, when in reality, adding details to a conjunction of events actually makes it less probable. The representativeness heuristic might severely bias the judged probabilities of detailed scenarios, such as those described to represent pathways to nuclear war or nuclear terrorism (see Chapter 4).

Probability Neglect

The perception of risk and avoidance behavior is roughly as strong when the probability is very small (but not zero) as when it is quite high (Rottenstreich and Hsee 2001). Sunstein (2003) observed that, when probability neglect is at work, people's attention is focused on the bad outcome itself, and they are inattentive to the fact that it is unlikely to occur. When consequences carry sharp and strong affective meaning, as is the case with a lottery jackpot or a cancer, the variation in probability often carries too little weight. As Loewenstein and colleagues (2001) observe, one's images and feelings toward winning the lottery are likely to be similar whether the probability of winning is 1 in 10 million or 1 in 10,000. They further note that responses to uncertain situations appear to have an all-or-none characteristic that is sensitive to the possibility rather than the probability of strong positive or negative consequences, causing very small probabilities to carry great weight. This perception helps explain why societal concerns about such hazards as nuclear power and exposure to extremely small amounts of toxic chemicals fail to recede in response to information about the very small probabilities of the feared consequences from such hazards. Rottenstreich and Hsee (2001) show that if the potential outcome is emotionally powerful (e.g., experiencing a painful electric shock), the strength of actions to avoid that outcome is relatively insensitive to changes in the probability of experiencing that outcome as great as from 0.99 to 0.01. Sunstein (2003) described this phenomenon as probability neglect and related it to expensive measures to reduce risks from terrorism that were extremely improbable.

Framing

There are often multiple ways to describe or frame the probability of an uncertain event. These descriptions can make a large difference in the perception of the risk and in subsequent decisions, even when they are logically identical (McNeil et al. 1982). For example, consider a man who is being evaluated for release from a hospital where he has been treated for a mental condition that posed a risk of violence. Is it safe to release him? Clinicians who are told that 1 in 10 persons like this individual are likely to be violent if released judge him as more dangerous and are less likely to release him than are clinicians who are told that 10 percent of persons like him are likely to be violent (Slovic et al. 2000). The frequency frame evokes images of "the guy being violent" that do not occur as often with a percentage frame.

Although this example shows that different representations of the same probability can lead to different risk perceptions and decisions, the same can be true of different representations of the same event or consequence. This occurs because probability judgments may be attached not to events but to descriptions of events (Tversky and Koehler 1994). The more explicit the description, the more likely the event seems. For example, in one study, the mean judgment of the probability of a death in the United States occurring from an *unnatural cause* was about 70 percent higher when participants were asked to estimate and then sum separate probabilities for each of these components of unnatural causes: accidents, homicides, or other unnatural causes. After describing numerous examples of this phenomenon, Tversky and Koehler concluded that probability judgments can be like the measured length of a coastline which increases as the map becomes more detailed. This highlights a major problem with probability assessments, namely, the need to consider unavailable possibilities. This problem is likely to be especially difficult when dealing with new hypotheses or the construction of novel scenarios, such as those discussed below.

While experience and rational reasoning are critical for expert judgment, many biases can distort intuitive judgments. An early overview of such cases was presented by Kahneman and colleagues (1982) and updated and extended by Kahneman (2011). Some methods for decreasing judgmental biases focus on structuring the elicitation, including the following:

- Specifying the problem to define precisely what is being addressed;
- Identifying the variables of interest, including objectives, courses of action, consequences, and associated probabilities and uncertainties;
- Selecting experts with substantial expertise in different parts of the risk analysis and a wide range of credible views on the parameters or events of interest;
- Facilitating the communications among experts so that they can exchange their mental models as well as their base of experience;
- Designing and pilot testing the elicitation process and questions;
- Training experts—for example, explaining the desired response format (such as percentiles)—and educating them about overconfidence and other biases;
- Processing the elicited data—for example, by performing sensitivity analysis or providing feedback to the experts; and
- Avoiding imposing accountability indiscriminately, since some accountability amplifies rather than attenuates bias (Lerner and Tetlock 1999).

Even with these approaches, there are problems with expert judgment that may not be addressed adequately. It has been known for many years that modest levels of training and feedback may not significantly reduce overconfidence in estimating the precision of one's estimate of an uncertain quantity (Moore 2020; Moore and Healy 2008). For example, a study by Alpert and Raiffa (1982) found that after one round of feedback, "The percentage of times the true values [being estimated] fell outside the extreme values (i.e., the 0.01–0.99 confidence ranges) fell from a shocking 41% to a depressing 23%" (Alpert and Raiffa 1982, p. 324). A more effective strategy is the use of "intensive performance feedback" (Lichtenstein and Fischhoff 1980; Plous 1993). However, that process can be burdensome both for the experts whose opinions are being assessed and for the risk analyst performing the assessment. The items used for training in one context may not generalize to other contexts, and expertise in a particular discipline may not translate into expertise on how best to express what an expert knows in probabilistic terms (Fischhoff et al. 1978).

Cooke (1991) developed a method for aggregating expert judgments based on the performance of the experts on "seed questions" with answers that are known (e.g., the extent of radioactive deposition observed in a tracer experiment) or knowable (e.g., prices of company stocks or real estate in the next month). The Cooke method, which evaluates expert judgments using scoring rules (to lessen the chance of experts gaming the system), has been applied in diverse fields, including medicine, maintenance, banking, real estate, nuclear safety, volcanology, food safety, and climate change, and was accepted by the UN Compensation Commission as an adequate basis for assessing the reparations due from Iraq to Kuwait for the Kuwaiti oil fires in the early 1990s (over $50 billion) (Cooke and Goossens 2008). The Cooke method frequently puts zero weight on some subset of the experts whose opinions were assessed, because their performance on the seed questions was demonstrably much poorer than that of other experts in the same study. Lin and Bier (2008) found significant differences in the extent of overconfidence among experts in a given study, lending support to the differential weighting of experts. Similarly, Cooke and Goossens (2008) indicate that in the majority of studies, performance weighting yielded better calibration than equal weights, and it also yielded better calibration than the judgment of the best-calibrated individual expert (Cooke and Goossens 2008).

This approach has several advantages. It does not generally require great statistical knowledge on the part of the experts whose opinions are being elicited. Moreover, Aspinall (2010, p. 295) wrote: "The speed with which such elicitations can be conducted is one of their advantages. Another advantage is that it encourages experts wary of getting involved in policy advice: the structured, neutral procedure, and the collective nature of the result, reassures experts and relieves them of the burden of sole responsibility." The Good Judgment Project (Mellers et al. 2014; Tetlock and Gardner 2015), established in response to a competition by the Intelligence Advanced Research Projects Agency, has taken a roughly similar approach, using empirical data to help identify the best-performing forecasters. This body of work has found that some people are much better than others at providing probabilistic forecasts of future geopolitical events, even though many of them had no specialized training or formal expertise. In fact, such well-calibrated laypeople (known as "superforecasters") often outperform intelligence experts with access to classified intelligence (McKinley 2021).

This finding means that, even though some experts can be biased, there is evidence that empirical calibration of expert opinion is feasible and can produce useful results. It thus seems appropriate to combine structuring elicitation with empirical calibration to improve the information obtained from expert elicitation. Indeed, Sutherland and Burgman (2015, p. 317) observe that "a large and growing body of literature describes methods for engaging with experts that enhance the accuracy and calibration of their judgments." Additionally, it should be noted that specific training tools for debiasing judgment have been developed by Morewedge and colleagues (2015).

Calibration of multiple experts can be difficult when the experts have different sources of information: therefore, it is important, if possible, to understand the basis of their opinions. Nuclear war and nuclear terrorism pose a multiple-expert challenge because of the different character, amount, or quality of the information available to different experts, as well as a spectrum of political viewpoints.

Laypeople who have been shown empirically to be well calibrated can provide a useful and relatively unbiased source of input, even without access to classified information. A technical expert may also assess knowledge of adversary capability and intent without any access to intelligence data. An analyst may have access to many intelligence sources that provide information on political, social, and economic aspects of capability and intent, but still may not understand the details of adversary technological capabilities or limitations. And a senior intelligence analyst may have access to information provided by very sensitive intelligence sources and methods that are not available to the broader intelligence community. Care should be taken to assess the value of different sources of input objectively, without excessive deference to seniority or access to classified information, since that can bias the results of an analysis.

The judgmental biases in many situations of nuclear war and nuclear terrorism may be quite different from those in other elicitation problems, raising serious challenges for these methods, notably because of the lack of direct experience with modern versions of either hazard and the strong emotions associated with events and their consequences. Efforts will be needed to develop and validate methods for making expert elicitations adequately trustworthy in these contexts.

ASSUMPTIONS IN RISK ANALYSIS

Technical and Modeling Assumptions

Technical and modeling assumptions are inevitably part of any risk analysis, including the definition of the risk problem and the conditions under which the analysis is expected to be valid. Some assumptions may have to be made to account for unavailable information, others may have to be made for the convenience or simplification of a particular model or analysis technique, and some may have to be made to suggest a particular course of action. Such assumptions are often necessary, and it is important for policy makers and other stakeholders to be aware of these assumptions since they can affect the applicability and reliability of risk analyses.

Modeling assumptions can include presumptions about adversaries (discussed below in more detail), about the reliability of data, and about the future evolution of technical systems. They may also be needed to simplify otherwise overly complex models. These assumptions are sometimes based on the conclusions of prior studies or analyses, which introduce additional levels of uncertainty. Other times, they may be well-established facts and historical events and behaviors that demonstrate the possibility that a particular kind of event can still occur. Nevertheless, it has to be demonstrated that they have relevance for future events. As described in Chapter 6, the very act of describing the risk events that go into a model is an exercise of judgment that carries implicit values that may strongly affect the analysis (Slovic 1999).

Technical assumptions, including the operational capabilities of various weapons (e.g., their reliability, survivability, precision, and effects) or the capabilities of detectors (e.g., false-alarm rates, failure to provide an alarm, sensitivity and standoff distances of radiation detectors) are involved in the analysis of many questions related to the risks of nuclear war and nuclear terrorism. Many of these assumptions may be reasonably well understood or characterized through testing or detailed modeling and may even be codified within a given agency or service so that all analysts are using the same data or assumptions. Such technical assumptions, sometimes called planning factors, play an important role in risk analyses related to nuclear war and nuclear terrorism. These technical assumptions, however, have to be revisited when the system is modified or the geopolitical situation has changed.

It is important to note that unidentified assumptions are a serious source of error in risk analysis. Such assumptions can include, for example, that the systems will operate as designed, that the intended processes are captured appropriately in the models, and that no oversimplifications or systemic biases exist.

Assumptions About Adversaries

Assumptions about adversaries may be necessary for risk analyses related to nuclear war and nuclear terrorism, but specifying realistic assumptions is not always straightforward. Rationality can be defined as the quality of preferences (are they reasonable by a given set of standards?) or by the consistency of their actions in aligning with their preferences (the von Neumann–Morgenstern preference axioms). In the latter case, some preferences of the adversary can be internally consistent but unacceptable by the given standards of morals and ethics. Uncertainty exists when making assumptions about both aspects of rationality.

Adversarial risk assessment in a game analysis has to make assumptions about the capability, goals, information, intent, and behavior of specific adversaries. It is typical for analyses of adversarial risks to assume at least some degree of consistency on their part. This assumption may be appropriate for some types of stable adversaries and stable circumstances (e.g., nation states or organized terrorist groups, although their preferences can change), but less appropriate for other adversaries, such as lone-wolf or other terrorist actors, who may be more opportunistic or idiosyncratic in their choice of targets and attack strategies, or apocalyptic terrorist groups, who are not attempting to achieve a set of goals.

What is rational and consistent to one adversary may be misunderstood or simply overlooked by another. Stable adversaries may change their arsenals and their strategy, and past actions may not be representative of future moves. Regimes can change and circumstances can change, so the nature of a conflict can be affected suddenly. The cognitive, social, and political biases described by Slovic and Lin (2020) challenge and explore the assumptions of rationality and consistency of all actors (Slovic et al. 2020). Adversaries can also act irrationally or signal that they would act irrationally if provoked. In some cases, the irrationality of an adversary may go beyond the bounded rationality of human cognition and extend into delusional or insane patterns of thought.

Assumptions About the Reliability of Data

Risk analysts may also make assumptions about the reliability and accuracy of the data available to them. For example, judgments from the intelligence community (e.g., National Intelligence Estimates) may be taken as givens, despite the risk that these judgments may be biased, inaccurate, or incomplete. The lack of experience with nuclear war and nuclear terrorism implies that risk analyses will have to rely extensively on multiple sources of information, including technical models and tests, surrogate data, historical experience, and expert opinion. This is especially challenging in assessing the risks of nuclear war or nuclear terrorism because of the consequences of such attacks.

Assumptions to Simplify Complex Models

Risk analysts often make assumptions to simplify an otherwise complex model and its formulation. It is important to be aware of such assumptions, to ensure that they are valid, and to understand how they might color the results. A fully realistic model could be as complex as the world it is trying to represent. The challenge is to make sure that simplifying assumptions do not ignore or obscure phenomena that are critical to the risks being analyzed.

Examples of simplifying assumptions that may be inappropriate in an analysis include treating uncertain quantities as if they were known, assuming probabilistic independence (that the occurrence of one event does not change the likelihood of other events), and presuming that the magnitudes of effects are proportional to those of causes. In reality, nonlinearities can mean that a small change in one element produces a large consequence.

Another factor that may be overlooked in complex dynamic situations is the possibility that seemingly favorable events could actually increase the risk of a particular event, while apparently unfavorable events could decrease it. For example, it might seem natural that a more sensitive detector would be more useful than a less sensitive one, but it is possible that increased sensitivity leads to an increase in false alarms, the consequence being that the problematic detector is turned off or ignored. Thus, an attempt to improve security instead diminishes it. Yet a sensor that is not sensitive enough might miss an event altogether or leave little lead time to react to a signal. Managing this tradeoff and deciding what is the best warning threshold to reduce the identified risk is one of the challenges of risk management (Paté-Cornell 1986).

U.S. STRATEGIC ASSUMPTIONS ABOUT NUCLEAR RISKS

U.S. assumptions are developed by analysts and decision makers, often as starting points for further analysis. These assumptions are often not explored by those conducting risk analysis, though they may serve to define the boundaries or constraints of a given analysis (OSD 2018).[3] Therefore, the connection between strategic assumptions about risks and the analysis of the risks of nuclear war or nuclear terrorism can be unclear, implicit, or tenuous in some cases. Understanding assumptions provides a context for the types of questions that should be asked of risk analysts by decision makers.

To make the rationale for its policies clear, the United States communicates many of the assumptions that underlie its nuclear security strategy in publicly available documents.[4] Given this commitment, many strategic assumptions are explicit in U.S. nuclear security strategy policy and documentation, and they are diverse in character from general assumptions about the nature of deterrence to specific assumptions about the goals of particular nuclear nations, potential proliferators, and nonstate actors. Some of these assumptions are explicit about risks related to nuclear war and nuclear terrorism, such as assumptions about whether certain policies or actions have increased or decreased risks, the nature and variety of threats that confront the United States, and the most likely scenarios.

The committee has identified the following five key categories of strategic assumptions that enter into risk analysis for nuclear war and nuclear terrorism:

- Assumptions about the risks posed by nuclear weapons use,
- Assumptions about the strategic intent of adversaries,
- Assumptions about the capabilities of and information available to adversaries,
- Assumptions about U.S. strategic goals, and
- Assumptions about deterrence.

These assumptions are often made explicit through assertions in public statements or other documents. A sampling of U.S. government statements on assumptions associated with nuclear risks is shown in Appendix A.

---

[3] Modeling assumptions, discussed above, are developed and used by those conducting risk analysis and are different from strategic assumptions.

[4] Those documents include the Nuclear Posture Review, National Security Strategy or Strategic Guidance, National Strategy for Countering Weapons of Mass Destruction Terrorism, and the Annual Threat Assessment of the U.S. Intelligence Community, among many others.

CONCLUSIONS

CONCLUSION 5-1: Information elicited from experts is often all that is available for assessing some aspects of the risks associated with nuclear war and nuclear terrorism. Analysts and decision makers need to be aware of the sources of that information, of the biases and limitations that the experts could introduce in the analysis, and of the resulting effects of this information on the results of risk analyses. Best practices for expert elicitation can be adapted from other risk analysis disciplines, although some aspects of nuclear war and nuclear terrorism may pose challenges in applying these methods.

CONCLUSION 5-2: Analysts inevitably make assumptions in risk analysis, including about the definition and framing of the risk problem; which models can be used effectively; the reliability of the available data; and the capabilities, intent, and potential actions of adversaries. It is important to show and clearly communicate assumptions and related uncertainties in a risk analysis and their effect on the results.

CONCLUSION 5-3: Strategic assumptions can affect the characterization of a risk problem. Some strategic assumptions address the nature or magnitude of risks, the effect of risk drivers, whether policies or actions increase or decrease the risks, the nature and the variety of threats that confront the United States, and the most likely scenarios. Strategic assumptions also concern risks of nuclear wars outside the borders of the United States.

6

Risk Analysis Methods and Models

Both quantitative and qualitative analytic methods can play a role in assessing specific components of the risks related to nuclear terrorism and nuclear war. While the analysts who are assessing the overall risks of nuclear war and nuclear terrorism are confronted by significant uncertainties related to lack of direct evidence; complex interdependencies; and changing technologies, policies, and geopolitical context, more narrowly defined risk problems may be more valuable to decision makers.

Risk analysis includes identification of risk management options and analysis of the effect of these options on the base risks. It is outside of the statement of task of this committee to analyze the policy or launch decisions that can be made by the decision makers. However, risk assessments can provide useful information to better inform decision makers.

Often, the questions that confront decision makers involve risks related to components of the overall risks, in particular risks associated with the country's own systems or capabilities. Such questions might involve scenarios about which a great deal is known and may therefore be more tractable than assessing overall risks. These kinds of questions might include, for example:

- Do communications in the command-and-control system of nuclear forces work as intended (Paté-Cornell and Neu 1985)?
- What is the reliability of a particular country's nuclear stockpile?
- What is the probability that a particular model of detector at an automobile border crossing will detect a specific level of radiation (with probabilities of false positives and false negatives)?

- How quickly does a particular material used in a nuclear weapon degrade?
- Which nuclear facilities should be inspected and how often?

Such questions might be addressed qualitatively, by structuring the understanding of the system, or quantitatively, by assigning probabilities to the events or failure modes identified in that risk structure. Some risk analyses are based on a combination of models that address both deterministic and probabilistic variables. Analyses often involve integrated models that select the most appropriate technique for each part of the risk analysis process—such as a reliability analysis of a system or subsystem, probability of detection of a sensor suite, the reliability of a communications network or the dynamics of external events. The choice of specific techniques is determined in part by the decisions that the risk analysis is intended to inform, the availability of relevant input, and the desires of the decision maker regarding the form of the results.

OVERVIEW OF METHODS

Table 6-1 briefly summarizes common analysis methods that have been or could be used for assessing the risks of nuclear war and nuclear terrorism. (For more detailed discussions of selected methods for both likelihood and consequence assessments, see Scouras et al. 2021.) In addressing a particular question, analysts may draw on multiple methods and many sources of evidence. This table relies only on publicly available information and is not intended to be exhaustive.

Note that some of the models presented in this table have not yet been applied to nuclear war and nuclear terrorism or published in the open literature. They are presented here as analytical options that can be used to assess the risks. It is important for all models to be validated prior to their use. This can be a time-consuming process but is essential for reliable implementation in any setting.

FIRST-STRIKE STABILITY ANALYSIS

First-strike stability analysis uses models and simulations to examine the nuclear capabilities that would remain on both sides if one side were to carry out a preemptive nuclear strike on the other side and vice versa. These analyses are conducted over a range of possible attacks spanning adversaries and their capabilities (e.g., their weapon systems and alert statuses). The results from these analyses can inform operational and logistical decisions, such as determining options for storing and protecting resources, evaluating possible force structures and alert statuses, assessing different strategic arms control agreement options, and planning scenarios for specific attacks. In particular, these analyses provide a starting point for evaluating response options by each side following the initial strike—a situation that becomes more complex as additional nuclear states develop capabilities and numbers that bring them closer to parity with the current nuclear superpowers.

Many methods can be brought to bear to feed first-strike stability analyses with information. Common examples are drawdown curves, which can be as simple as a representation of remaining blue force weapons after red attacks of varying size. These depend on assumptions about aggressor and defender capabilities and give insight into what aggressor and defender capabilities exist following a first strike. Other factors that could be considered include how preemptive actions could result in destabilizing actions from adversaries (e.g., creating new weapon technologies to counter the reinforcement of existing weapon silos) and how actions can cascade in a multi-actor scenario.

PROBABILISTIC RISK ASSESSMENT

Probabilistic risk analysis (PRA) (also known as probabilistic safety analysis) provides an analytical structure and yields quantitative results. Originally developed for nuclear power plants (NRC 1975), it has been developed further to include human and management errors, as well as the dynamics of systems (e.g., deterioration) and the evolution of external events (e.g., environmental factors). Yet, like all quantitative methods of risk analysis, it can contain large uncertainties and dependencies on underlying assumptions. These uncertainties are reflected to some degree in the resulting risk curves (probability distributions of outcomes), but additional representations are needed to describe the uncertainties in the probabilities and their effects in the results. Functional diagrams, fault trees, event trees, influence diagrams, and dynamic stochastic models are used to represent the underlying structure. When extending a risk analysis to a decision analysis, decision points and approaches are introduced in the model to better understand the inherent uncertainties associated with different options.

The first step in a PRA is to characterize the functions of the system, and which ones are essential to the success of its operations, as well as the external events that affect the reliability of the different components. This is done through a functional diagram representing system functions in series or in parallel and through event trees or fault trees (Paté-Cornell 2009).

Fault trees are often used to identify failure modes when analyzing the failure probabilities of engineered systems (Aven 2008; Rausand and Hoyland 2003), but they are not generally necessary for other kinds of systems. Event trees are based on the specification of events contributing to the considered outcome (e.g., total failure of the system). They include probabilities and dependencies to provide the probabilities of the different scenarios based on the failure modes, thus a probability distribution of the outcomes (Paté-Cornell 1984). As noted above, PRA has evolved considerably since its introduction in 1974—now including, for instance,

TABLE 6-1 Risk Analysis Methods

Method	Applicability and Strengths	Limitations	Examples of Use for Risks of Nuclear War or Nuclear Terrorism
First-Strike Stability Analysis	This method compares the surviving nuclear forces of both actors for the two cases in which (1) one actor attacks the nuclear forces of the other side first, and (2) the other actor strikes first.	This method is limited to the contribution of force structure and posture to incentives to strike first in a crisis; it ignores myriad other relevant factors.	This method can be used to evaluate different force structures and alert statuses. It can also be used to assess different strategic arms control agreement options. Resources: Cimbala and Scouras (2002); Scouras (2019)
Probabilistic Risk Assessment (PRA)	PRA was originally developed for engineered systems but has been applied to other fields and to interactions between intelligent adaptive actors and other nontechnical risk analyses. PRA provides an analytical structure and yields quantitative results with quantified uncertainties. Classical statistics and Bayesian probabilities can be used to reflect uncertainties in available information.	The major challenges of applying PRA to the risks of nuclear war are identifying the scenarios, and assessing their probabilities and consequences. These probabilities have to be communicated to decision makers in a way that they understand, recognizing that it can be challenging to grasp and represent the complex structure and functions of a system and the interactions among actors. While the quantitative results from PRA can be converted into qualitative results, nuance can be lost in the process.	The Department of Homeland Security has used PRA to assess the risks of nuclear terrorism. PRA can be used to analyze terrorist pathways to nuclear weapons use and potential defender responses. It can be used to evaluate the risks associated with defender capabilities, acquisition of materials, production of sufficient material, weaponization of that material, reliability of technical systems involved in nuclear weapons maintenance and signal communication, transportation to the target area, final deployment at the target, exposure and other effects of nuclear weapons use, ability of the public health system to provide effective medical countermeasures, and potential human health and economic consequences from an attack. Resources: Paté-Cornell and Guikema (2002); Paté-Cornell and Neu (1985)
Order-of-Magnitude Estimates	An order-of-magnitude estimate provides a simplified framework for estimating overall risks for nuclear war and nuclear terrorism. This begins with upper and lower bounds, which are then incrementally decreased and increased respectively until a range of values is identified that cannot be ruled out easily.	This intuitive approach is subject to the challenges typical of expert elicitation. This approach has not yet been widely tested.	Resources: Hellman (2011); Scouras et al. (2021)

continued

TABLE 6-1 Continued

Method	Applicability and Strengths	Limitations	Examples of Use for Risks of Nuclear War or Nuclear Terrorism
Nuclear Effects Simulation	Built on mathematical models, deterministic or probabilistic simulations use data (e.g., weapons yield, weather condition, wind speed) to estimate effects of nuclear weapons.	Nuclear effects simulation models are based on available test data and the nature of many long-term effects that are not well known. The resolution and accuracy of these models vary.	These simulations can be used in war games involving nuclear terrorism or limited use of nuclear weapons. Resources: Bele (n.d.); Nasstrom et al. (2007)
Game Theoretical Approaches	Game theory, or game analysis, is a standard approach for situations with intelligent adversaries.	Game theory analysis is limited by the knowledge of what the adversaries know, want, and have. Representing these limitations is critical to the value of the results. As with probabilistic methods, uncertainties are introduced in the analysis and represented in the results.	Game theory was arguably the basis for the mutually assured destruction policy during the Cold War. Resources: Brams (2001); Ice et al. (2019); Kucik and Paté-Cornell (2012); O'Neill (1994); Schelling (1960, 1980)
Adversarial Risk Analysis (ARA)	ARA can be used to model the strategic choices of an intelligent opponent. It might apply to situations in which one has a small number of actors and fairly accurate knowledge about the goals, capabilities, and decision making of those actors. The model also includes uncertainties—for example, those represented by Bayesian probabilities.	ARA may be more effective in modeling scenarios with a small number of actors (e.g., a nuclear threat by North Korea against the United States), but it would not be easy to use when assessing the possible actions of opportunistic terrorists.	ARA is relatively new, but older versions of the method have been applied in the context of game analyses. ARA has not been directly used in many complex settings. As an extension of game analysis, however, it has been used to model and simulate counterterrorism policies, considering alternative decisions of a government and a terrorist group. Resources: Banks et al. (2015); Rios Insua et al. (2012)

Agent-Based Models	Agent-based models are based on rules that determine the interactions among actors. They can also reflect uncertainties of each actor about the motivations and potential responses of others to actions of the actor.	These models can be difficult to identify and validate as the rule sets may change over time. It is difficult to test the goodness-of-fit of agent-based models for particular applications since relevant statistics are seldom available. The models should include uncertainties relevant to the decisions made by the actors and the interaction rules.	Some attempts have been made to apply agent-based models to understand approaches to deter the development and use of nuclear weapons. Resources: Banks and Hooten (2021); Carley et al. (2018)
Multi-Attribute Models	Multi-attribute models specify the key attributes of the preferences of an actor and then assess the behavior of actors that pose the largest risk.	These models rely on expert opinions from policy and intelligence experts.	These models have been used by the Sandia National Laboratories global risk and decision analysis team. Resources: Bauer et al. (1999); Caskey and Ezell (2021); Caskey et al. (2018)
Network Models	Network models use network analysis to explore multiple alternatives at nodes representing key events and scenarios in the path from start to end. These models can be deterministic or probabilistic and used to identify the shortest path to a given outcome, which can help focus intelligence resources.	General cases may be difficult to address depending on the description of scenarios. As applications become more complex and the options multiply, the combinatorial complexity makes these methods more difficult to use. Their implementation depends on the analysts' computational capabilities.	Network models can be used to assess the nuclear capability of a nation state or terrorist organization from program start to operational readiness. These models are useful in thinking through a set of specific nuclear threats and risk scenarios. Resources: Freeman (2010); McIntosh and Storey (2018)

continued

TABLE 6-1 Continued

Method	Applicability and Strengths	Limitations	Examples of Use for Risks of Nuclear War or Nuclear Terrorism
Nuclear Force Exchange Models	Nuclear force exchange models can be used to assess the potential effectiveness of nuclear attacks and can be part of a first-strike stability analysis. These models can use weapon-specific technical information (e.g., planning factors) to estimate nuclear force capabilities.	These model outputs depend on users developing possible attack strategies, potentially imbedding biases or inaccurately reflecting relevant scenarios.	These models have been used to assess conflict scenarios, such as the North American Trade Organization vs. Warsaw Pact, North Korea, and variations of bilateral compared with trilateral arms agreements. Resource: Hafemeister (2014)
Conventional Force Models	Conventional force models can be used to assess the potential effectiveness of conventional force attacks. These models can be used to compare the effectiveness and consequences of a conventional force attack with a nuclear attack. These models can use weapon-specific technical information to estimate conventional force capabilities.	These model outputs depend on users developing possible attack strategies, potentially imbedding biases or inaccurately reflecting relevant scenarios. The variety of conventional weapons and possible scenarios compound these challenges.	These models are used broadly to assess potential conflict scenarios. Resources: Ali et al. (2007); Betts (1985); Larson (2019); Stockfish (1975)

a system's evolution and deterioration, as well as the human and organizational errors that affect the failures of the system components or constitute failure modes in themselves (Murphy and Paté-Cornell 1996).

In more detail, a combination of fault trees and event trees can be used to characterize the reliability of a system. Fault trees are constructed using inductive or top-down logic starting with a hypothesized failure or undesired event (the top event) and working backward to identify the combinations of basic events that could give rise to that top event. In the context of this report, the top event might be a successful terrorist attack on a nuclear plant, and the basic events could be a forcible breach of plant security or the radicalization of an employee. A fault tree includes a logic diagram that shows Boolean representations of the basic components (i.e., by two values—for example, by true or false, or by 0 or 1, happens or not), as well as the Boolean relationship between the basic events and the top event (a system or subsystem failure) and the possible causes of that event (the sets of component failures called failure modes). The tree itself represents how the states of the system's components (basic events) relate to the state of the system as a whole, using logic gates. Probabilities are then used to assess the chances of the different failure modes and of failure of the system.

A detailed fault tree might involve numerous events or be decomposed to examine the role of each subsystem in a system's failure. The failure modes (minimum combinations of component failures leading to system failure) can be identified from the logical functions of the fault tree. The probability of the top event can then be computed as a function of the probabilities of these failure modes, accounting for the effects of external events and the human errors that may affect the failure probabilities of several components and subsystems. To construct the fault tree itself, one needs a description of the system's function, which is provided by a functional block diagram. Boolean results allow for the identification of failure modes, whose probabilities can then be assessed to yield the chances of the top event (system failure). In technical systems, fault trees allow identification of the combinations of events and the Boolean variables (0 or 1) that constitute the failure modes. Once the failure modes have been identified, one can compute their probabilities, including dependencies and external events.

Event trees are deductive (in contrast with fault trees) and based on random events and random variables and their probability distributions (Paté-Cornell 1984). The results of a fault tree analysis and the probabilities of failure modes can be included in an event tree to assess the probability distribution of different possible outcomes (including system failure, or a range of losses in a successful terrorist attack). Event trees are widely applicable to analyses of a spectrum of scenarios, including terrorist nuclear attacks). They are constructed using deductive logic. The process may start by hypothesizing the initiating event of a failure scenario, such as terrorists' acquisition of fissile material or an alarm indicating the possibility of an incoming intercontinental ballistic missile. It then works forward to identify all possible combinations of subsequent events (whether successes, failures, or multi-outcome results) and their probabilities, conditional on what precedes them in the tree, to determine which combinations of events would lead to undesirable outcomes and their probabilities. WASH-1400 (NRC 1975), one of the first applications of PRA to an engineered system, introduced fault trees and event trees in the nuclear technical realm. Dynamic models representing an anticipation of future evolutions, both of systems and of the external events that affect their operations, are now part of PRAs and especially relevant to the assessment of nuclear risks.

An event tree represents the events following an initiating event and decomposes the scenarios by showing all possible pathways to outcomes. For example, risk analysts in the Department of Homeland Security use an event tree methodology when analyzing potential nuclear terrorism attack scenarios. Monte Carlo simulation, based on the generation of random values of different events and factors and the functions in which they appear, can be used to generate multiple realizations of a given loss function and provide a final set of likelihoods and consequences realizations for the set of scenarios. Similarly, the National Nuclear Security Administration noted in communication to the committee that knowledge about nuclear devices and pathways to their development allows the overall probability of a given scenario to be decomposed into probabilities of acquisition, processing, fabrication, and use of nuclear materials in an analysis of risks. "Since there may be higher confidence in one of these terms over another, the partitioning approach enables resources to focus on improving the quantification of those terms where the greatest uncertainty or highest potential for impact to a risk assessment may exist, and subsequently redirect USG [U.S. government] efforts after achieving an acceptable level of confidence."[1]

The combination of fault trees and event trees is useful when considering technical systems because their functions can be combined to provide a final risk result. Event trees are useful if one wants to display the chronological order of events and the dependencies among uncertain factors. The events in an event tree do not have to be in chronological order. The probabilities on any branch are conditioned on the realizations of the random variables that precede the events in the tree regardless of the timing. Their order can thus be chosen as a function of the structure of the information available. Event trees therefore display dependencies among events (e.g., if the quality of emergency response depends on environmental conditions). This type of dependency is readily apparent since the failure probabilities of each component or occurrences of various events are shown on the relevant branches. For these reasons, event trees are good for facilitating communication about the

[1] L. Leonard, Department of Homeland Security, "Response to NASEM Questions on DHS Risk Assessments," Washington, DC, September 15, 2021.

effects of the assumptions made in the risk model. However, because both successes and failures are explicitly shown and can have more than two realizations, event-tree models can rapidly become extremely large.

Fault and event trees are used to develop a probability distribution of the consequences of the scenarios. The probabilities of the output quantity of interest (e.g., losses) reflect the uncertainties of individual component failures. Event trees include both systematic (epistemic) and random (aleatory) uncertainties in the form of marginal or conditional probabilities: see Appendix B for more discussion of these types of uncertainties. While they are included in event-tree analysis, systematic (epistemic) uncertainties—for example, those resulting from disagreements among experts or imperfect knowledge—can be separately described to a decision maker, and the effect of these uncertainties can be assessed, through such methods as a sensitivity analysis. This is important as the two types of uncertainty have different implications for decision making. Although aleatory uncertainty cannot be reduced (e.g., the result of the roll of the dice), a high level of systematic (epistemic) uncertainty may imply that more research or intelligence gathering might be desirable (if feasible) before deciding about options for risk reduction. Yet it should be understood and communicated that more information may actually *increase* uncertainties—for example, if a new failure mode is discovered in the process of a risk analysis—which may be an important consideration for the decision maker.

As noted above, these methods are often used to analyze the failure probabilities of outcomes, including failure of particular systems or subsystems, both technical and social. These methods have been applied in many fields, including nuclear power plants, aerospace systems such as the space shuttle, chemical and petrochemical facilities, and medical procedures. They can even support qualitative analysis: for example, Barrett and colleagues (2013a) use a simplified fault tree representation to structure an analysis of inadvertent nuclear war.

While the general form of a probabilistic risk assessment for nuclear power plants today is not dramatically different from that used in the *Reactor Safety Study* (NRC 1975), substantial improvements in methodology have been developed to enable the method to handle more complex and realistic situations. But many nuclear threat scenarios are quite complex, and the application of probabilistic risk assessment may be difficult.

Risk analysis seeks to identify the actions that minimize the expected loss. When there is both great uncertainty about the probabilities of events and the magnitude of the consequences, probabilistic risk assessment will represent these uncertainties as probability distributions of outcomes based on the limited information available. Yet, one should recognize that some decision makers may have difficulties relating these probabilities to the decisions that they have to make, and that both the analytical methods and the results have to be carefully explained.

ORDER-OF-MAGNITUDE ESTIMATES

One intuitive approach to assessing the overall probability of nuclear war, proposed by Hellman (2011), can generate results with a wide range of uncertainty. Hellman briefed the committee on his approach, which begins by considering an extreme case: a probability of 1 percent per day. He argues that this is clearly too high; in his words, "we would not expect to live out the next year." By the same token, a probability of 1 in 1,000,000 per year is, in his view, clearly too small. Hellman then argues for increasing the lower bound and decreasing the upper bound, an order of magnitude at a time, until a range of values is identified that cannot easily be ruled out. He argues that even an estimate covering two orders of magnitude of uncertainty can be policy relevant.

Hellman uses historical events such as the 1962 Cuban missile crisis and adaptations of expert elicitation to develop his intuitive estimate that the probability of nuclear war is 1 percent per year to an order of magnitude. While the method described above does not constitute a PRA, as described in this report, Hellman suggests that some form of PRA of the overall risks of nuclear war could be used to further develop the rough probabilities into estimates of overall risks of nuclear war, albeit with large uncertainties (Scouras et al. 2021).[2]

This intuitive approach merits further investigation as a means to estimate the overall risks for nuclear war. It has not yet been widely tested.

NUCLEAR EFFECTS SIMULATIONS

Nuclear effects simulations use mathematical and statistical models to estimate the effects of nuclear weapons. These simulations can help inform the understanding of how a detonation would impact a particular location, which can inform decision making. However, these simulations can contain large uncertainties because they often depend on sparse real-world data and a limited understanding of many long-term effects.

While these simulations can be designed to account for many types of effects, they often combine location-specific information (e.g., buildings, populations, transit systems) with the anticipated effects from a detonation (e.g., the blast wave, intense heat, radiation, and radioactive fallout) to estimate the total impact. Longer-term effects, such as the toll on human social, emotional, and physical health, as well as the long-term economic costs resulting from cleanup and rebuilding, are less well understood and so difficult to include.

---

[2] The policy use of risk estimates with very large uncertainties is a more appropriate subject for Phase II of this study, which will examine the interplay between the result of risk analyses and national security strategy more directly.

This type of information can be helpful for scenario planning, but it is not generally well suited for precise calculations of impacts.

GAME THEORETICAL APPROACHES

Increasingly, analyses require some model of an adversary. Such analyses depend on both the characteristics and actions of users and attackers.

Approaches that involve multiple decision makers, typically adversaries, can be understood as games against one or more adversaries (Paté-Cornell 2009; Schelling 1960). Such approaches often focus on questions with uncertain answers: What do the adversaries know? What do they want? What do they have? Information to address these questions can come from a variety of open sources as well as the intelligence community and other experts.

Game theoretical approaches can be conducted qualitatively, which approach allows identification of the various options available to the different sides under variable circumstances, based on expert opinions. The task is to identify (qualitatively) the moves that are most likely to be chosen by other sides, without quantitative support of the probabilities and consequences of the different scenarios or of the preferences of the decision makers. The doctrine of mutually assured destruction that prevailed during the Cold War is one example of the use of qualitative analysis, along with the quantification of scenarios and options.

Quantitative game theory has been used in security studies (Bier 2005; Bier and Azaiez 2008; Bier et al. 2007; Zhuang and Bier 2007), and quantitative game analysis methods can include behavioral games, as well as games on hierarchical and nested networks. A key component of these models is the response of each side to a move from another. The model is thus dynamic and allows simulation of the long-term effects of a defense policy or strategy by modeling the alternative actions of both sides (Kucik and Paté-Cornell 2012). Network theory, and influence diagrams in particular, thus plays an important role in this context, as it represents explicitly the formal notion of interaction. The use of networks and influence diagrams implies fundamental insights about interactions, which are sparse, have different strengths, can be directed or asymmetric, and can vary in time.

MODELING OF ADVERSARIES

Explicit Bayesian Modeling

Modeling an opponent is something human beings do regularly, either implicitly or explicitly. In the domain of counterterrorism, a Bayesian model of the effectiveness of policy from a government to interdict or counter the actions of a terrorist group was constructed based on two influence diagrams representing the decision of each of the two sides at each time unit in a determined time horizon (Kucik and Paté-Cornell 2012). The model was applied to the counterinsurgency measures of the Philippine government faced with a terrorist group in the island of Mindanao with input from the U.S. Army and the Philippine Army. It was then used to simulate the effects of chosen paths at each time by each side over 3 years, and the results for that time period were compared to the actual situation. Bayesian modeling of opponent interactions is thus possible on a similar pattern for nuclear conflicts between nations, but it is likely to be more difficult, given the uncertainties involved, when trying to model organized multinational terrorist organizations.

Other game analyses involving several actors that act over time can be constructed on a similar pattern, but with different assumptions (e.g., not only rationality in the classic economic sense) regarding the preferences of the different sides.

Adversarial Risk Analysis

Adversarial risk analysis (ARA) is an alternative to classical game theory that uses Bayesian subjective distributions to model the goals, resources, beliefs, and reasoning of the opponent. In this framework, subjective probability distributions can be used for all unknown quantities, which results in a distribution over the opponent's actions that accounts for uncertainty. While ARA reduces the need for common knowledge, it can be computationally expensive (Banks et al. 2022).

ARA is relatively new, but older versions of the method have been applied in the context of game analyses. ARA may be more effective in modeling scenarios with a small number of opponents (e.g., a nuclear threat by North Korea against the United States), but it would not be easy to use when assessing the possible actions of opportunistic terrorists.

OTHER MODELS

Agent-Based Models

Agent-based models study the behavior of systems of virtual entities that interact with each other and their environment according to prescribed rules. A classic example of these models is the principal-agent model, involving, for instance, a supervisor and a subordinate. The composed dynamics of agent interactions can be then used to study interesting patterns that one observes, while providing a certain amount of causal understanding (using rules of interaction) of why these patterns arise. Agent-based models have been used to explore cellular automata, interacting particle systems (Banks and Hooten 2021), and traffic flows on roadways (Barrett et al. 2002; Nagel et al. 1999). In this traffic model, the agents are endowed with multiple behavioral rules, including carrying out a daily itinerary, deciding modes of transportation, finding the best way to get to their destination, and driving on the road while avoiding accidents. In other words, the virtual vehicles interact with each other and their environment (e.g., the road network, the weather, and the time of day) according to rules that determine spacing, speed, route choice, and other factors.

In the context of nuclear threats and consequences, agent-based models can be developed to understand and assess risks for a nuclear event. The social, economic, and health impacts of an improvised nuclear device as a part of the national planning scenario can be also studied using agent-based models (Barrett et al. 2013c; Parikh et al. 2013). Agent-based models have also been developed to study the social, behavioral, and economic impact of the use of nuclear weapons (Swarup et al. 2013). Such a model might develop a detailed representation of a group of individuals or an organization, understand the pathways by which they can obtain fissile material, and represent intent and their ability to compute the consequences of their actions. In other words, one can build a rich representation of the underlying processes and constraints that might lead an organization/country to carry out a nuclear attack. However, the model's output depends on the factors considered and the completeness of that set. In addition, it would have to be mapped to a probability distribution, and this has been a significant challenge for agent-based models in general (Heard 2014). Agent-based models that forecast weather may be calibrated on the basis of their empirical accuracy, but there are almost no data that could be used to calibrate nuclear risks. In other words, while events, interactions, and consequences can be represented, the associated information and data to calibrate these models, validate the social theories, and quantify the uncertainty are challenging given the lack of statistical data. Additional challenges stem from the computational resources that would be required to couple models at different scale and fidelity. Additional information, including expert opinion, would then be needed to address this key aspect of the model.

Multi-Attribute Models

Multi-attribute models specify the key attributes of the preferences of a decision maker, such as a nuclear state or a nuclear terrorist group, and then assess their behavior that would cause the biggest risks to the United States or its allies. Each of these criteria may be weighted according to the perceived importance placed on them by the adversaries. Different objectives or possible actions may be in conflict with one another in a multi-attribute model. These models can be structured in many different ways, such as with multi-attribute utility functions (Bauer et al. 1999; Keeney and Raiffa 1976) or using an analytical hierarchy process (Andrews et al. 2008). Both deterministic and stochastic network models are used to estimate nuclear capabilities of nuclear states. Subject-matter experts, such as political scientists or intelligence experts, help define preferences of nuclear adversaries in order to populate these models to predict the behavior of high-risk terrorist groups.

Network Models

Influence diagrams (a generalization of Bayesian networks to include decisions) represent a decision analysis based on risk analysis; these often have the same fundamental inputs and outputs as event trees, but also include decision nodes and the value function of the decision maker. Like the Bayesian networks, they show the dependencies among random variables and events, as well as the resulting distributions of input and outcomes and the values attached to them by the decision maker. In both Bayesian networks and influence diagrams, the model has to include a set of numerical tables representing the dependencies among the factors and the resulting distribution of the consequences, as well as the diagram. As the system evolves and the risks change, stochastic processes representing that evolution need to be introduced in the analysis.

Pathway Models

Pathway and network models are used to identify the potential activities that an adversary could perform to obtain a nuclear weapon or delivery system. They can represent multiple variables and decision nodes in the pathway to a user's decision and its consequences. For example, for nuclear weapons delivery systems, once the potential activities (paths) that an adversary could take are identified, intelligence systems can look for potential signals of these activities.

Network Analysis

Complex networks exist throughout society, including transportation and communication networks. Network science deals with principles that govern the design, analysis, control, and optimization of networks. Recent quantitative changes in computing and communications have created new opportunities for collecting, integrating, accessing, and analyzing information related to such networks, and these enhance analysts' ability to formulate, analyze, and implement policies pertaining to them. As networks become pervasive, they reduce the time it takes to transmit information between various agents or organizations. Furthermore, they introduce new connections between systems—together creating challenges for resilient decision making in the event a nuclear war or terrorist activity.

Real-world networks are large, heterogeneous, and evolve over time, and their dynamics, behavior, and network structure are interdependent. Reasoning, predicting, and controlling these networks are challenging because the dimension reduction techniques commonly used to analyze physical systems are difficult to apply.

Network analysis seeks to assess the relationships and interdependencies among connected entities. These approaches have been applied to problems related to nuclear and other forms of terrorism, as well as nuclear deterrence (Carley et al. 2018; Morgan et al. 2017) and the consequences of a nuclear explosion on the power grid (Barrett et al. 2013b). Much like agent-based models, dynamic multilevel network analysis can be used to represent sensor networks for detecting the movement of nuclear material (Cazalas 2018; Srikrishna et al. 2005) or to identify central actors that might be involved in the exchange of nuclear material or information.

Nuclear Force Exchange Models

Nuclear force exchange models can approximate the potential effectiveness of a nuclear attack by estimating the expected physical damage, including pre-launch survivability, in-flight survivability, weapon reliability, and probability of damage (incorporating factors such as accuracy, yield, and height at burst). While some of these models are deterministic with one expected outcome, most are probabilistic and provide a range of possible outcomes that depend on the given force structure and other characteristics. Some analyses use input from a variety of models and resources, including submodels that capture detailed phenomena about known variables (e.g., missile trajectory, detonation reliability, blast impact characteristics), as well as existing damage calculators that are used across organizations.

These models can be used as part of a first-strike stability analysis or as a standalone assessment of the risks of a nuclear attack.

Conventional Force Models

Like nuclear force exchange models, conventional force models can be used to assess the potential effectiveness of conventional force attacks, accounting for known variables and uncertainties and yielding deterministic or probabilistic outcomes. However, the abundance of available conventional weapons and the expanded delivery options greatly expand the possible modeling scenarios. Mission planning and other decisions are also complicated by the plethora of factors and options. It is important to note, however, that only some weapons and systems are assumed to affect nuclear stability.

Relative Risk

Relative risk expresses the differences in risk among a set of scenarios or mitigation strategies. This kind of assessment uses some of the methods described above to frame risk information in a way that may be more understandable and thus more useful to decision makers. However, to compute relative risks, one generally has to start from the value of an absolute risk, then assess the effects of changing the values of the relative factors.

Artificial Intelligence and Nuclear Risks

Artificial intelligence (AI)[3] is a rapidly developing technology that is revolutionizing the analysis of large datasets and is being widely explored in military and intelligence applications, with particular interest in its support of fast decision making (Schmidt et al. 2021). Associations identified by AI systems are typically based on empirical correlation and they can offer unexpected insights into the relationships between variables. However, they can also produce results that are profoundly biased or simply incorrect (e.g., CRS 2021; Kumar et al. 2019). Because only limited data are available, decision making regarding a nuclear crisis and the use or threat of the use of nuclear weapons may not be well suited for AI.

In the case of deep learning, the processing typically includes nonlinear steps, such as thresholding, whereby variables are downweighted or completely dropped if their values lie outside certain ranges. Correlations can develop in unanticipated and nonlinear ways, with small perturbations resulting in large changes during the analysis. In contrast with many traditional pattern-recognition processes that are linear and can be run backward and undone, processing nonlinearities can effectively prevent deep-learning algorithms from being reversed in order to understand what determines the outcome. The availability of massive amounts of computer processing has been an asset for AI, but also serves as a liability because of increased reliance on cloud and edge computing, which create opportunities for adversary exploitation (CRS 2021; West and Allen 2020).

However, there are at least two types of nuclear-relevant applications in which AI might be implemented to varying degrees to support nuclear decision making: surveillance, warning, and reconnaissance; and communications (Hruby and Miller 2021). The use of AI in an adversarial manner, to challenge human analysis and judgment in wargaming and related activities intended to improve crisis management, could be another helpful role for AI systems.

[3] AI primarily refers to machine learning, including such approaches as supervised or reinforcement learning and deep learning; see CRS (2021) and West and Allen (2020) for brief, nontechnical summaries.

AI continues to evolve rapidly, and much effort is being made to use physics, as well as insights from the behavioral and social sciences, to improve AI results. However, progress along these lines has been surprisingly difficult, and many of the failures are still poorly understood. Pressures for rapid decision making, as well as the lack of relevant training examples, increase these vulnerabilities of AI, as do the challenges for appropriate interfacing between human and machine-based decision making. The lack of transparency and accountability compound these risks.

CONCLUSION

CONCLUSION 6-1: Different methods of risk assessment are more or less well suited for different situations and goals. For risk management problems that involve significant uncertainties and a need to make resource-constrained decisions, assessing the risk variations associated with different options can help inform decision making. The results of relative risk assessments may be more useful and easier to communicate to a decision maker than the absolute risk.

7

Risk Information and Risk Management Decisions

Just as the structure, parameters, and modeling assumptions in a risk analysis may affect the results, the formulation of the risk analysis and the communication of risk information affects decision making. This chapter addresses some of what is known about human judgment and decision making under uncertainty and the communication of the results of risk analyses.

EMPIRICAL STUDY OF JUDGMENT AND DECISION MAKING

The dawn of the nuclear age coincided with new academic interest in understanding how people make judgments and decisions, including those involving risks. Economists and other scientists developed decision analysis models, guiding decision making based on the analysis of outcomes and uncertainties. At the same time, psychologists, political scientists, and philosophers began to conduct experiments asking people to make judgments and decisions about simple gambles to study how people make decisions under uncertainty and in the face of risks.

Normative models of decision making have long been dominated by theories that described how rational people choose among options. Faced with uncertain or risky prospects, the option that has the highest *expected value* or *expected utility* (when values were expressed as utilities based on individual preferences and risk attitudes) is expected to be chosen. Moreover, a decision maker's preferences are assumed to be orderly; for instance, someone who preferred option A over option B and option B over option C is expected to prefer option A over option C.

Early cognitive theorists and experimentalists were skeptical of the accuracy of these views and instead focused on descriptive models. Herbert Simon's (1957) influential book *Models of Man* introduced the notion of *bounded rationality* that took human cognitive limitations into account. He proposed that people actually search for solutions that are "satisfactory" rather than "optimal," and stop searching when the first satisfactory solution is found.

Experimental psychologists were even more skeptical than Simon about the accuracy of the expected utility approach. Their studies found preference patterns that could not easily be accounted for by economic theory (Coombs and Pruitt 1960; Edwards 1953, 1954). Edwards's work motivated others to study decisions across a wide range of everyday human activities, including medical diagnoses and treatments, and technologies, such as nuclear power and chemicals. New fields of study were created (e.g., risk perception) along with a new conception of choice that recognized that many of human's most important decisions are determined by preferences that are constructed during the act of deciding (Jasanoff 1986; Lichtenstein and Slovic 2006; Slovic 1995). These constructed preferences are very much influenced by subtle contextual factors, such as the way the choice options are framed or described and the specific nature of the response.

The instability inherent in observed preferences was radically different from prevailing notions of rationality (Gretter and Plott 1979). Half a century after the beginning of this movement, Daniel Kahneman received the 2002 Nobel Memorial Prize in economics for his research with Amos Tversky (who had died in 1996) on the psychology of risk and decision making, leading to a new discipline called behavioral economics.

Preference instability is likely to be especially prevalent in situations in which decision makers' values have not been shaped by learning from experience or for which there have been no events and, thus, no experience. It poses a challenge for theories of nuclear deterrence that assume rational preferences and for risk assessment methods that rely on understanding the values and preferences of experts and decision makers.

Group judgment of risks has also been explored with respect to decision making under uncertainty. Contrary to the "two heads are better than one" idiom, risk assessment by a group of people that are interacting directly with each other is not necessarily better than individual judgment and can be worse (Houghton et al. 2000). Not only do heuristics and biases guide individual judgment and decision making under uncertainty, but they also play a role in group judgments and decisions. In groups, individual judgments can be affected by biases such as groupthink and information pooling (Stasser and Titus 1985; Turner and Pratkanis 1998). Group biases have been at least partly to blame for such incidents as the USS *Vincennes* mistaking a civilian airbus for a pending enemy attack in 1988 (Johnston et al. 1998), and for the decisions made leading to the 1986 *Challenger* shuttle disaster

(Hughes and White 2010). Similarly, mistakes at the group level can also be made in the course of communicating risk assessment to decision makers.

The *Vincennes* incident prompted a large research program on tactical decision making under stress. This program resulted in team training and technology solutions aimed at facilitating group judgment and decision making and avoiding biases (Cannon-Bowers and Salas 1998). As an example of a technological mitigation, Rajivan and Cooke (2018) demonstrated that information visualizations to improve perceptual processing and memory in the cyber security domain could reduce the information pooling bias. That is, the visualization facilitated the sharing of information held uniquely by individuals (Stasser and Titus 1985). Professional facilitators have developed practices to improve group judgment and decision making and to avoid group bias (Bens 2017; Kaner 2014; Schwarz 2002). For instance, facilitators are trained to support group judgment and decision making by testing assumptions; asking questions; and paraphrasing, summarizing, and synthesizing ideas (Bens 2017). For judgments and decisions on issues as consequential as nuclear war and nuclear terrorism, it would be of value to consider some of these mitigation procedures.

An evolving area of research on judgment and decision making concerns emotion and risk analysis (Slovic 1999). The field of emotion science has grown substantially in recent years. Relevant to the perception of terrorism and of nuclear war, research has shown predictable relationships from specific emotions and risk perception, some of which are very counterintuitive (Lerner et al. 2015). For example, although anger is a negative emotion (which intuition suggests should produce a negative outlook), anger actually diminishes the perception of risks (e.g., Ferrer et al. 2017; Lerner and Keltner 2001). A nationally representative study revealed that anger and fear have opposing effects on risk perception: fear increases the perceived risks of terrorism, and anger decreases such perceptions (Lerner et al. 2003). As understanding of the ties between emotion and risk perception have become better understood, the inclusion of motivation has also entered into the field (Lerner et al. 2015; Phelps et al. 2014).

Few decision makers would experience neutral emotion in the context of a nuclear attack, and so models need to be infused with specific parameters predicting the effects of emotions on the depth of information processing, on implicit goal activation, and on the content of information processing (Lerner et al. 2015; Phelps et al. 2014). In addition, it is important to recognize that high-stakes decision making occurs in the context of social and institutional systems with norms, culture, and systems of accountability.

Studies of the ways people make decisions and the logical problems associated with intuitions have challenged assumptions of rationality. The question is whether risk analysis and the notion of rationality can help address these behavioral problems, especially when policies and decision making involve the management of the risks of nuclear war and nuclear terrorism.

THINKING ABOUT RISKS

While social scientists were conducting experiments to understand the cognitive dynamics of heuristics and biases in judgments under uncertainty, and the fundamental nature of preference and choice, societal disagreements were emerging over such topics as the safety of nuclear power plants and pesticides. At the heart of these conflicts was the perception of risks and safety (Covello et al. 1986; Starr 1981), and questions regarding the sensitivity of judgments to some characteristics of risks, such as controllability, equity, and unstated uncertainties (Slovic 1987).

Subsequent analyses contested the distinction between objective and subjective risks, arguing that assessing risks is thoroughly subjective, based on (1) theoretical models whose structure is subjective; (2) assumptions; (3) inputs that are dependent on judgment, from the initial structuring of a risk problem to deciding which endpoints or consequences to include in the analysis; and (4) identifying and estimating exposures to the hazard (Slovic 1999). Even the apparently simple task of choosing a risk measure for a well-defined endpoint such as human fatalities can be surprisingly complex and judgmental.

For example, there are many different ways that fatality risks from exposure to a toxic chemical can be described and measured, including but not limited to (Slovik 1999)

- Deaths per million people in the population
- Deaths per million people within *x* miles of the source of exposure
- Deaths per unit of concentration
- Deaths per facility
- Deaths per ton of air toxin released
- Deaths per ton of air toxin absorbed by people
- Deaths per ton of chemical produced
- Deaths per million dollars of product produced
- Loss of life expectancy associated with exposure to the chemical

An analyst has to select which measures to use in a risk assessment, recognizing that the choice could make a big difference in how the risks are perceived and evaluated.

Recent research about thinking has clarified new ways of understanding decision making. While early studies of risk perception were primarily descriptive, more recent research has benefited from theoretical advances in cognitive psychology that inform the underlying mechanisms that drive perceptions and behavior. In particular, dual-process theories (e.g., Epstein 1994; Finocchiaro 1994) distinguish between what Kahneman later characterized as fast and slow thinking (intuitive or analytical decision making) (Kahneman 2011).

According to these theories, people apprehend reality in two fundamentally different ways: "fast" is intuitive, automatic, natural, nonverbal, narrative, and experiential; "slow" is analytical, deliberative, and verbal. Note that although the latter is likely to be slower if the analysis takes time, rational thinking may also be intuitive and quick. Fast thinking, which may be nonconscious, relies on intuition, quick impressions, reflexive judgments, and gut feelings. Slow thinking relies on careful analysis and deliberation, often with numbers and calculations. People rely on fast thinking most of the time because it is easier and feels right in spite of frequent mistakes in understanding uncertainties, as described by Tversky and Kahneman (1974). Education, however, may lead some to slow down, to think rationally through uncertainties rather than accepting their first intuitive conclusion.

Risk analysis is designed to help those who wish to think more systematically about decisions characterized by danger and uncertainty, and to avoid some of the mistakes known to compromise the rationality of such decisions. It is a relatively recent tool in the long evolution of analytical thinking. From the origins of mankind, human brains developed the capacity to think symbolically, and apply logic and reason to guide decision making beyond immediate instincts. Analytical thinking enables one to imagine and critically evaluate consequences of actions beyond those "right in front of our eyes." It is important for decision makers to recognize the need to think rationally, and make the effort to do so, especially when the potential consequences of the decisions are extreme, outside the realm of direct experience, or when external events, such as a changing geopolitical situation, can drastically affect the risks.

Misinformation and disinformation are real and ongoing threats. The committee did not discuss or explore the role of this threat as it pertains to risk analysis; it may be addressed in the second phase of the committee's work.

Clearly, human intuitions about risks and uncertainties can be wrong in significant ways, and human decision making can be deeply flawed. Risk analysis, when conducted as objectively and transparently as possible to support decision making (rather than to justify an already-made decision), can inform decision makers and stakeholders, and enhance their ability to make decisions with a clear understanding of the available information and its implications.

COMMUNICATING RISK ANALYSIS RESULTS

Risk analysis is conducted to inform decisions and policies. Therefore, the findings of these analyses must be communicated effectively to those who need to use them. The difficulties people have in understanding risks point to the need to train analysts and decision makers to communicate risk information in ways that are cognizant of how people think about and understand risks. An individual's mental model, or approach of thinking about a problem, can also have a significant effect on how the results are interpreted (Morgan et al. 2002).

Research has shown that the presentation of risk information is a *frame* that can greatly influence the way the information is interpreted and used. For example, probabilities can be expressed (i.e., framed) quantitatively as numbers between 0 and 1, as percentages, or as relative frequencies. They can be expressed qualitatively through words such as unlikely, rare, or probable. Verbal probability, however, may be translated into a wide range of numerical probabilities by the receiver (Beyth-Marom 1982), and numerical and verbal probabilities used in risk assessments may not be equally accurate (Budescu et al. 2014).

Another example of a framing problem is that percentage and frequency formats are interpreted differently. For example, as mentioned above, a 1 percent (or 0.01) chance of a harmful event occurring tends to be seen as less risky than the logically equivalent chance of 1 in 100. The latter triggers mental images of the harmful event occurring ("imagining the numerator"), creating unpleasant feelings that increase the perceived risks. The 1 percent or 0.01 frames rarely produce such imagery, and thus create less feeling of a dangerous situation. Similarly, an event described as having a 90 percent chance of success may be perceived much more favorably than the same event described as having a 10 percent chance of failure (Slovic et al. 2000).

Framing problems can contribute to communication breakdowns. The 2011 nuclear accident at the Fukushima Daiichi Nuclear Power Plant is one such example. Since 2007, the frequency of a disaster-inducing tsunami at the plant has been estimated to occur approximately once every 1,000 years or less (Rampton 2011), or a 0.1 percent chance annually on average. The government and plant owner Tokyo Electric Power Company failed to frame the frequency of disaster events appropriately and to clearly communicate the risks to the public, resulting in unsatisfactory evacuation orders and poor emergency preparedness (Faculty of Societal Safety Sciences 2018). These missteps contributed to the eventual nuclear accident at Fukushima.

Another problem is that precise estimates or a lack of a discussion of uncertainty associated with likelihoods or quantities can be seen as more trustworthy than estimates surrounded by uncertainty bounds or presented as a range (Johnson and Slovic 1995; Van der Bles et al. 2019). An unfortunate corollary is that it may be tempting to hide these uncertainties from the decision maker, exactly when uncertainties should be an important part of a decision.

Although events whose likelihoods are certain or near certain may trigger a strong response, differences in less extreme probabilities may not matter much in the way people make decisions (Rottenstreich and Hsee 2001; Sunstein 2003). Context also matters. The word "rarely" may be interpreted much differently when referring to a disease than when referring to a hurricane, or a headache compared with blindness (Fischer and Jungermann 1996). And a scenario describing a possible disaster may be perceived as more likely when surrounded by text describing common but irrelevant information that contributes to the perceived reality of the scenario (Tversky and Kahneman 1983).

When sufficient data allow one to describe risks quantitatively, analysts face a wide choice of options regarding the specific measures and statistics used to communicate the magnitude of risks, as illustrated in the list above. In a similar vein, Wilson and Crouch (2001) used coal mining statistics to demonstrate how different measures of the same risks can sometimes create quite different impressions. They showed that accidental deaths per million tons of coal mined in the U.S. had decreased steadily over time. In this respect, the industry was getting safer. However, they also showed that the rate of accidental deaths per 1,000 coal mine employees had increased because the miners had become more productive. Neither measure was the one right measure of overall mining risks. They each told part of the same story.

Individuals' fluency with numerical information (numeracy) varies and greatly affects the degree to which one can draw appropriate meaning from quantitative information about risks and other important matters (Peters 2020). Political ideologies also skew the interpretation and response to technical information and analysis (Makridis and Rothwell 2020). Trust in the analysts and the communicator is also a major factor in how information is received and acted on. Trust is affected by the degree to which the communicator is perceived to share one's values and is acting in one's best interests. Messages sent from an opposing political party or based on a process that is not seen as fair or inclusive of diverse views may be distrusted and ignored (Flynn and Slovic 1993; Kahan et al. 2010).

Another key factor in the quality of communications is the choice of the language that is used in the interaction (e.g., quantitative or qualitative), as well as the decision maker's understanding of the sources of information and the way it was processed (Blastland et al. 2020; van der Bles et al. 2020). Having an intermediary explain to the consumers of the information the meaning and limitations of technical analyses can improve understanding.

It is difficult to predict how a risk analysis will be received without testing it in advance. While testing is challenging in times of conflict, different frames may be pretested on relevant audiences to identify potential problems in subsequent communication. Experts in communication can play important roles in ensuring that risk analyses are properly understood.

> The magnitude of the risks associated with nuclear and radiological weapons is inherently difficult to assess and communicate. It becomes even more problematic when descriptions of the weapons and their effects are communicated with what Cohn (1987) called tech-

> nostrategic language, or in terms that are abstract, euphemistic, and devoid of negative emotion. A review of the war games conducted by RAND in the 1950s noted that games with detached, quantitative, emotionless language, and devoid of moral judgment, were more likely to lead to the use of nuclear weapons than games with emotional realism and ethical considerations. (Emery 2021)

Risk analysis can be a key input to a risk management decision, but framing and communication of risk information also has an effect on the decision makers and the options they choose. Of course, the results of risk analyses are not the only—or sometimes even the most important—factors in decision making. Decisions involve, in addition to the risk results, the risk attitude and preferences of the decision maker.

CONCLUSION

CONCLUSION 7-1: The ways that risk information is assessed, framed, or presented have powerful effects on how that information is understood and used in decisions. Risk analysis results are most valuable when the method and assumptions by which they were generated is clear, the process is replicable, trust in the analytical process is established, and the analysis addresses the real questions or decisions that confront the decision makers.

8

Conclusions and Next Steps

This report explores the nature and the use of risk analysis methods to assess the risks of nuclear war and nuclear terrorism, based on unclassified information. In doing so, the report explores the structure of risk analysis, the history and literature of risk assessment for nuclear war and nuclear terrorism, and approaches to understanding the threat of nuclear war and nuclear terrorism.

This is the first in a two-part effort; the second phase will expand the focus to include an analysis of the role that the methods and assumptions in risk analysis may play in U.S. security strategy. This second phase is expected to produce a classified report, along with an unclassified summary.

New technologies, including in cyber and space domains, offer technical means to reduce the risks of—but also to provide new routes toward—crisis and conflict. Whether the overall risks are increasing or decreasing with time is unclear, but the uncertainties in the risks associated with nuclear conflict have been increasing over recent decades because of the emergence and broad dissemination of powerful new technologies, as well as a shift toward multipolar nuclear competition.

The committee reached 11 conclusions, as detailed in the preceding chapters.

CONCLUSION 3-1: The U.S. nuclear posture has evolved over time, taking into account new threats, developing deterrence strategies against different U.S. adversaries, technological advancements, nuclear arms reductions, and changing geopolitical environments. U.S. assessments of the risk of nuclear terrorism have likewise evolved over time, taking into account the new threats and emerging technologies.

CONCLUSION 4-1: There is a need to improve the understanding of less-well-understood physical effects of nuclear weapons (such as fires; damage in modern urban environments; electromagnetic pulse effects; and climatic effects, such as nuclear winter), as well as the assessment and estimation of psychological, societal, and political consequences of nuclear weapons use.

CONCLUSION 4-2: The U.S. government and the international community have invested significant resources and time in trying to understand and reduce the risks of nuclear war and nuclear terrorism. The risks remain real and are becoming more complex as new technologies and new adversaries arise.

CONCLUSION 4-3: There is a fundamental lack of direct evidence about nuclear war and nuclear terrorism. Analysts attempt to mitigate the resulting uncertainties by applying different methods and using multiple sources of information to supplement the limited body of evidence.

CONCLUSION 4-4: Assessing the overall risks of nuclear war and nuclear terrorism involves great uncertainties about the likelihood and consequences of different scenarios. The assessment and communications of these uncertainties are critical for policy decisions essential to managing these risks.

CONCLUSION 4-5: The value of risk analysis is not solely in assessing the overall risks of nuclear war or nuclear terrorism. Risk analysis can provide valuable input on many specific problems related to nuclear war and nuclear terrorism, including an understanding of the uncertainties involved.

CONCLUSION 5-1: Information elicited from experts is often all that is available for assessing some aspects of the risks associated with nuclear war and nuclear terrorism. Analysts and decision makers need to be aware of the sources of that information, of the biases and limitations that the experts could introduce in the analysis, and of the resulting effects of this information on the results of risk analyses. Best practices for expert elicitation can be adapted from other risk analysis disciplines, although some aspects of nuclear war and nuclear terrorism may pose challenges in applying these methods.

CONCLUSION 5-2: Analysts inevitably make assumptions in risk analysis, including about the definition and framing of the risk problem; which models can be used effectively; the reliability of the available data; and the capabilities, intent, and potential actions of adversaries. It is important to show and clearly communicate assumptions and related uncertainties in a risk analysis and their effect on the results.

CONCLUSION 5-3: Strategic assumptions can affect the characterization of a risk problem. Some strategic assumptions address the nature or magnitude of risks, the effect of risk drivers, whether policies or actions increase or decrease the risks, the nature and the variety of threats that confront the United States, and the most likely scenarios. Strategic assumptions also concern risks of nuclear wars outside the borders of the United States.

CONCLUSION 6-1: Different methods of risk assessment are more or less well suited for different situations and goals. For risk management problems that involve significant uncertainties and a need to make resource-constrained decisions, assessing the risk variations associated with different options can help inform decision making. The results of relative risk assessments may be more useful and easier to communicate to a decision maker than the absolute risks.

CONCLUSION 7-1: The ways that risk information is assessed, framed, or presented have powerful effects on how that information is understood and used in decisions. Risk analysis results are most valuable when the method and assumptions by which they were generated is clear, the process is replicable, trust in the analytical process is established, and the analysis addresses the real questions or decisions that confront the decision makers.

On the basis of these specific conclusions, the committee offers three overall conclusions.

1. *Past examples of nuclear war and nuclear terrorism are rare. As such, there is little direct evidence that can be relied on to make empirical estimates about the probability of either.*
2. *The scenarios that might lead to nuclear war and nuclear terrorism are numerous and involve many interdependent factors, and the assessment of their risks often depend on the capabilities, values, perceptions, and intentions of many experts and actors.*
3. *Different risk assessment methods are more or less suited to different situations and goals.*

References

Acton, J.M. 2018. "Escalation Through Entanglement: How the Vulnerability of Command-and-Control Systems Raises the Risks of an Inadvertent Nuclear War." *International Security* 43(1):56–99. https://doi.org/10.1162/ISEC_a_00320.

AEC (Atomic Energy Commission). 1957. *Theoretical Possibilities and Consequences of Major Accidents in Large Nuclear Power Plants.* WASH-740. Washington, DC: U.S. Nuclear Regulatory Commission.

Ali, S.A., H.J. Carlo, and V. Cesani. 2007. "Distributed Intelligent Simulation and Decision Support System for Battlefield Management." Pp. 884–889 in *Proceedings of the IIE Annual Conference and Expo 2007 - Industrial Engineering's Critical Role in a Flat World.*

Allison, G.T. 2004. *Nuclear Terrorism: The Ultimate Preventable Catastrophe.* New York: Times Books/Henry Holt.

Allison, G.T., and P. Zelikow. 1999. *Essence of Decision: Explaining the Cuban Missile Crisis*, 2nd ed. London: Longman.

Allison, G.T., R. Cote, Jr., R.A. Falkenrath, and S.E. Miller. 1996. *Avoiding Nuclear Anarchy: Containing the Threat of Loose Russian Nuclear Weapons and Fissile Material.* Vol. 12. Cambridge, MA: MIT Press.

Alpert, M., and H. Raiffa. 1982. "A Progress Report on the Training of Probability Assessors." In *Judgment Under Uncertainty: Heuristics and Biases*, D. Kahneman, P. Slovic, and A. Tversky, eds. Cambridge, UK: Cambridge University Press.

Andrews, W.L., M. Helfrich, and J.R. Harrald. 2008. "The Use of Multi-Attribute Methods to Respond to a Nuclear Crisis." *Journal of Homeland Security and Emergency Management* 5(1). https://doi.org/10.2202/1547-7355.1337.

Ansoff, H.I., W.W. Baldwin, D.J. Davis, N.M. Kaplan, P. Kecskemeti, and A. Wohlstetter. 1951. *Outline of a Study for the Plans Analysis Section.* Santa Monica, CA: RAND Corporation.

Argyris, N., and S. French. 2017. "Nuclear Emergency Decision Support: A Behavioural OR Perspective." *European Journal of Operational Research* 262(1):180–193. https://doi.org/10.1016/j.ejor.2017.03.059.

Arms Control Association. 2001. *U.S. Withdrawal from the ABM Treaty: President Bush's Remarks and U.S. Diplomatic Notes.* https://www.armscontrol.org/act/2002-01/us-withdrawal-abm-treaty-president-bush's-remarks-us-diplomatic-notes.

Apostolakis, G. 1990. "The Concept of Probability in Safety Assessments of Technological Systems." *Science* 250(4986):1359–1364.

ASIS (American Society for Industrial Security). 2015. *Risk Assessment.* Standard ANSI/ASIS/RIMS RA.1-2015. Approved August 3, 2015. https://webstore.ansi.org/preview-pages/ASIS/preview_ANSI+ASIS+RIMS+RA.1-2015.pdf.

Aspinall, W. 2010. "A Route to More Tractable Expert Advice." *Nature* 463(7279):294–295.

Aumann, R.J., M. Maschler, and R. Sterns. 1995. *Repeated Games with Incomplete Information.* Cambridge, MA: MIT Press.

Auserwald, D. 2017. "The Evolution of the NSC Process." In *The National Security Enterprise: Navigating the Labyrinth,* R.Z. George and H. Rishikof, eds. Washington, DC: Georgetown University Press.

Aven, T. 2008. "Assessing Uncertainties Beyond Expected Values and Probabilities." In *Risk Analysis.* Hoboken, NJ: Wiley.

Banks, D.L., and M.B. Hooten. 2021. "Statistical Challenges in Agent-Based Modeling." *The American Statistician* 75(3):235–242.

Banks, D.L., J.M. Rios Aliaga, and D. Rios Insua. 2015. "Simultaneous Games." In *Adversarial Risk Analysis.* New York: Chapman and Hall.

Banks, D.L., V. Gallego, R. Naveiro, and D. Ríos Insua. 2022. "Adversarial Risk Analysis: An Overview." *WIREs Computational Statistics* 14(1):e1530. https://wires.onlinelibrary.wiley.com/doi/abs/10.1002/wics.1530.

Barrett, C.L., K. Bisset, R. Jacob, G. Konjevod, and M. Marathe. 2002. "Classical and Contemporary Shortest Path Problems in Road Networks: Implementation and Experimental Analysis of the TRANSIMS Router." Pp. 126–139 in *European Symposium on Algorithms*, R. Möhring and R. Raman, eds. Berlin: Springer.

Barrett, A.M., S.D. Baum, and K. Hostetler. 2013a. "Analyzing and Reducing the Risks of Inadvertent Nuclear War Between the United States and Russia." *Science and Global Security* 21(2):106–133. https://doi.org/10.1080/08929882.2013.798984.

Barrett, C.L., S. Eubank, C.Y. Evrenosoglu, A. Marathe, M.V. Marathe, A. Phadke, J. Thorp, and A. Vullikanti. 2013b. "Effects of Hypothetical Improvised Nuclear Detonation on the Electrical Infrastructure." Pp. 1–7 in *International ETG-Congress 2013; Symposium 1: Security in Critical Infrastructures Today.* https://ieeexplore.ieee.org/document/6661633.

Barrett, C.L., K. Bisset, S. Chandan, J. Chen, Y. Chungbaek, S. Eubank, Y. Evrenosoğlu, et al. 2013c. "Planning and Response in the Aftermath of a Large Crisis: An Agent-Based Informatics Framework." Pp. 1515–1526 in *Proceedings of the 2013 Winter Simulations Conference.* https://doi.org/10.1109/wsc.2013.6721535.

Bauer, K.W., G.S. Parnell, and D.A. Meyers. 1999. "Response Surface Methodology as a Sensitivity Analysis Tool in Decision Analysis." *Special Issue: Sensitivity Analysis in MCDA* 8(3):162–180.

Becker, S.M. 2012. "Psychological Issues in a Radiological or Nuclear Attack." Pp. 171–194 in *Medical Consequences of Radiological and Nuclear Weapons*, Department of Defense, ed. Washington, DC: U.S. Government Printing Office.

Bele, J.M. n.d. "Nuclear Weapons Effects Simulator and Models." *Nuclear Weapons Education Project.* https://nuclearweaponsedproj.mit.edu/nuclear-weapons-effects-simulator-and-models.

Bellinger, J. 2021. "National Security Memorandum 2—What's New in Biden's NSC Structure." *Lawfare* (blog). February 8. https://www.lawfareblog.com/national-security-memorandum-2-whats-new-bidens-nsc-structure.

Bens, I. 2017. *Facilitating with Ease! Core Skills for Facilitators, Team Leaders and Members, Managers, Consultants, and Trainers.* Hoboken, NJ: John Wiley and Sons.

Betts, R. 1985. "Conventional Deterrence: Predictive Uncertainty and Policy Confidence." *World Politics* 37(2):153–179. https://doi.org/10.2307/2010141.

Beyth-Marom, R. 1982. "How Probable Is Probable? A Numerical Translation of Verbal Probability Expressions." *Journal of Forecasting* 1(3):257–269.

Biden, J.R. 2021a. "Memorandum on Establishing the Fight Against Corruption as a Core United States National Security Interest." June 3. https://www.whitehouse.gov/briefing-room/presidential-actions/2021/06/03/memorandum-on-establishing-the-fight-against-corruption-as-a-core-united-states-national-security-interest.

Biden, J.R. 2021b. "Memorandum on Renewing the National Security Council System." February 4. https://www.whitehouse.gov/briefing-room/statements-releases/2021/02/04/memorandum-renewing-the-national-security-council-system.

Bier, V.M. 2005. "Game-Theoretic and Reliability Methods in Counter-Terrorism and Security Modern Statistical and Mathematical Methods in Reliability: Series on Quality." In *Reliability and Engineering Statistics*. Singapore: World Scientific Publishing Co.
Bier, V.M., and M.N. Azaiez, eds. 2008. "Game Theoretic Risk Analysis of Security Threats." Vol. 128 of *International Series in Operations Research and Management Science*, F.S. Hillier, ed. New York: Springer Science and Business Media.
Bier, V.M., and S.-W. Lin. 2013. "On the Treatment of Uncertainty and Variability in Making Decisions About Risk." *Risk Analysis* 33(10):1899–1907. https://doi.org/10.1111/risa.12071.
Bier, V., S. Oliveros, and L. Samuelson. 2007. "Choosing What to Protect: Strategic Defensive Allocation Against an Unknown Attacker." *Journal of Public Economic Theory* 9(4):563–587.
Binninger, G.C., P.J. Castleberry, Jr., and P.M. McGrady. 1974. *Mathematical Background and Programming Aids for the Physical Vulnerability System for Nuclear Weapons*. Washington, DC: Defense Intelligence Agency.
Blastland, M., A.L.J. Freeman, S. van der Linden, T.M. Marteau, and D. Spiegelhalter. 2020. "Five Rules for Evidence Communication: Avoid Unwarranted Certainty, Neat Narratives, and Partisan Presentation; Strive to Inform, Not Persuade." *Nature* 587:362–364. https://www.nature.com/articles/d41586-020-03189-1.
Blitzer, W. 2003. "Search for the 'Smoking Gun.'" January 10, 2003. *CNN*. https://www.cnn.com/2003/US/01/10/wbr.smoking.gun.
Bloembergen, N., C.K.N. Patel, P. Avizonis, R.G. Clem, A. Hertzberg, T.H. Johnson, T. Marshall, et al. 1987. "Report to the American Physical Society of the Study Group on Science and Technology of Directed Energy Weapons." *Reviews of Modern Physics* 59(3):S1–S201. https://doi.org/10.1103/RevModPhys.59.S1.
Bradley, M.M. 2007. "NARAC: An Emergency Response Resource for Predicting the Atmospheric Dispersion and Assessing the Consequences of Airborne Radionuclides." *Journal of Environmental Radioactivity* 96(1–3):116–121. https://doi.org/10.1016/j.jenvrad.2007.01.020.
Brams, S.J. 2001. "Game Theory and the Cuban Missile Crisis." *Plus: Bringing Mathematics to Life* (blog). January 1, 2001. Millennium Mathematics Project. University of Cambridge. https://plus.maths.org/content/game-theory-and-cuban-missile-crisis.
Brodie, B., ed. 1946. *The Absolute Weapon: Atomic Power and World Order*. New York: Harcourt, Brace and Co.
Buch, B., and S.D. Sagan. 2013. "Our Red Lines and Theirs: New Information Reveals Why Saddam Hussein Never Used Chemical Weapons in the Gulf War." *Foreign Policy* (blog). December 13, 2013. https://foreignpolicy.com/2013/12/13/our-red-lines-and-theirs.
Buddemeier, B. 2010. "Reducing the Consequences of a Nuclear Detonation: Recent Research." *The Bridge* 40(2):28–38.
Budescu, D.V., H.-H. Por, S.B. Broomell, and M. Smithson. 2014. "The Interpretation of IPCC Probabilistic Statements Around the World." *Nature Climate Change* 4(6):508–512.
Bukharin, O. 1996. "Security of Fissile Materials in Russia." *Annual Review of Energy and the Environment* 21(1):467–496.
Bundy, M., and S. Rosenblum. 1989. "Danger and Survival: Choices About the Bomb in the First Fifty Years—Review. *International Perspectives* 18(3):29–30.
Bunn, M. 2000. *The Next Wave: Urgently Needed New Steps to Control Warheads and Fissile Material*. Washington, DC: Carnegie Endowment for International Peace.
Bunn, M. 2006. "A Mathematical Model of the Risk of Nuclear Terrorism." *Annals of the American Academy of Political and Social Science* 607:103–120.
Bunn, M. 2013. *Beyond Crises: The Unending Challenge of Controlling Nuclear Weapons and Materials*. St. Louis: Federal Reserve Bank of St. Louis.
Bunn, M. 2021. "Twenty Years After 9/11, Terrorists Could Still Go Nuclear." *Bulletin of the Atomic Scientists* (blog). https://thebulletin.org/2021/09/twenty-years-after-9-11-terrorists-could-still-go-nuclear.
Bunn, M., and E. Harrell. 2014. *Threat Perceptions and Drivers of Change in Nuclear Security Around the World: Results of a Survey*. Cambridge, MA: The Project on Managing the Atom, Belfer Center for Science and International Affairs. https://www.belfercenter.org/publication/threat-perceptions-and-drivers-change-nuclear-security-around-world-results-survey.
Bunn, M., and D. Kovchegin. 2018. "Nuclear Security in Russia: Can Progress Be Sustained?" *Nonproliferation Review* 24(5–6):527–551.
Bunn, M., and N. Roth. 2017. "The Effects of a Single Terrorist Nuclear Bomb." *Bulletin of the Atomic Scientists* 28.

Bunn, M., and S.D. Sagan, eds. 2017. *Insider Threat*. Ithaca, NY: Cornell University Press.

Bunn, M., M.B. Malin, N.J. Roth, and W.H. Tobey. 2016. "Appendix: Evolving Perceptions of the Threat of Nuclear Terrorism." In *Preventing Nuclear Terrorism: Continuous Improvement or Dangerous Decline?* Cambridge, MA: The Project on Managing the Atom, Belfer Center for Science and International Affairs. https://www.belfercenter.org/publication/preventing-nuclear-terrorism-continuous-improvement-or-dangerous-decline.

Bunn, M., N. Roth, and W.H. Tobey. 2019. *Revitalizing Nuclear Security in an Era of Uncertainty*. Cambridge, MA: Belfer Center for Science and International Affairs.

Bush, G.W. 2001. "Organization of the National Security Council System." In *National Security Presidential Directive-1*. Washington, DC: The White House.

Butler, R. 2001. *Fatal Choice: Nuclear Weapons: Survival or Sentence*. Council on Foreign Relations. Boulder, CO: Westview Press.

Caffrey, M. 2000. "Toward a History-Based Doctrine for Wargaming." *Aerospace Power Journal* Fall:33–56.

Campbell, K.M. 1991. "The US–Soviet Agreement on the Prevention of Dangerous Military Activities." *Security Studies* 1(1):109–131.

Cann, M., J. Parker, and K. Davenport. 2016. *The Nuclear Security Summit: Accomplishments of the Process*. Washington, DC: Arms Control Association.

Cannon-Bowers, J.A., and E. Salas. 1998. "Team Performance and Training in Complex Environments: Recent Findings from Applied Research." *Current Directions in Psychological Science* 7(3):83–87.

Carley, K.M., G.P. Morgan, and M.J. Lanham. 2018. "Deterring the Development and Use of Nuclear Weapons: A Multi-Level Modeling Approach." *The Journal of Defense Modeling and Simulation* 15(4):483–493.

Caskey, S.A., and B. Ezell. 2021. "Prioritizing Countries by Concern Regarding Access to Weapons of Mass Destruction Materials." *Journal of Bioterrorism and Biodefense*. https://www.osti.gov/servlets/purl/1831169.

Caskey, S.A., A. Williams, and B. Ezell. 2018. *Use of Multi Attribute Decision Analysis Models to Characterize the WMD Vulnerabilities of Countries to Help Support Global Threat Reduction Actions*. Albuquerque, NM: Sandia National Laboratories. https://www.osti.gov/servlets/purl/1576892.

Cazalas, E. 2018. "Defending Cities against Nuclear Terrorism: Analysis of a Radiation Detector Network for Ground Based Traffic." *Homeland Security Affairs* 14(10). https://www.hsaj.org/articles/14715.

Chandan, S., S. Saha, C. Barrett, S. Eubank, A. Marathe, M. Marathe, S. Swarup, and A.K.S. Vullikanti. 2013. "Modeling the Interaction Between Emergency Communications and Behavior in the Aftermath of a Disaster." In *Social Computing, Behavioral-Cultural Modeling and Prediction*, N. Agarwal and K. Xu, eds. Vol. 7812 of *Lecture Notes in Computer Science*. Cham: Springer.

Cimbala, S.J., and J. Scouras. 2002. *A New Nuclear Century: Strategic Stability and Arms Control*. Westport, CT: Greenwood Publishing Group.

Clemen, R.T., and R.L. Winkler. 1999. "Combining Probability Distributions from Experts in Risk Analysis." *Risk Analysis* 19(2):187–203.

Cohn, C. 1987. "Sex and Death in the Rational World of Defense Intellectuals." *Signs: Journal of Women in Culture and Society* 12(4):687–718.

Colson, A.R., and R.M. Cooke. 2017. "Cross Validation for the Classical Model of Structured Expert Judgment." *Reliability Engineering and System Safety* 163:109–120.

Cooke, R.M. 1991. *Experts in Uncertainty: Opinion and Subjective Probability in Science*. Oxford: Oxford University Press on Demand.

Cooke, R.M., and L.L.H.J. Goossens. 2008. "TU Delft Expert Judgment Data Base." *Reliability Engineering and System Safety* 93(5):657–674.

Coombs, C.H., and D.G. Pruitt. 1960. "Components of Risk in Decision Making: Probability and Variance Preferences." *Journal of Experimental Psychology* 60(5):265.

Cornell, C.A. 1968. "Engineering Seismic Risk Analysis." *Bulletin of the Seismological Society of America* 58(5):1583–1606.

Covello, V.T., P. Slovic, and D. Von Winterfeldt. 1986. "Risk Communication: A Review of the Literature." *Risk Abstracts* 3:171–182.

CRS (Congressional Research Service). 2021. *Artificial Intelligence: Background, Selected Issues, and Policy Considerations*. Washington, DC: Congressional Research Service.

Crutzen, P.J., and J.W. Birks. 2016. "The Atmosphere after a Nuclear War: Twilight at Noon." Pp. 125–152 in *Paul J. Crutzen: A Pioneer on Atmospheric Chemistry and Climate Change in the Anthropocene.* Vol. 50 of *Springer Briefs on Pioneers in Science and Practice: Nobel Laureates*, H.G. Brauch, ed. Cham: Springer.

Cunningham, F.S., and M.T. Fravel. 2019. "Dangerous Confidence? Chinese Views on Nuclear Escalation." *International Security* 44(2):61–109.

Daly, S., J. Parachini, and W. Rosenau. 2005. *Aum Shinrikyo, Al Qaeda, and the Kinshasa Reactor: Implications of Three Case Studies for Combating Nuclear Terrorism.* Santa Monica, CA: RAND Corporation.

Danzig, R., A.M. Saidel, and Z.M. Hosford. 2012. *Beyond Fukushima: A Joint Agenda for US-Japanese Disaster Management.* Washington, DC: Center for a New American Security.

de Finetti, B. 1974. *Theory of Probability: A Critical Introductory Treatment.* Hoboken, NJ: Wiley.

Desmond, W.J., N.R. Zack, and J.W. Tape. 1997. *The First 50 Years: A Review of the Department of Energy Domestic Safeguards and Security Program.* https://www.osti.gov/biblio/562556.

DHS (Department of Homeland Security). 2017. *Instruction Manual 262-12-001-01.* DHS Lexicon Terms and Definitions, revision 2. October 16. https://www.dhs.gov/sites/default/files/publications/18_0116_MGMT_DHS-Lexicon.pdf. Original publication. September 2010. https://www.dhs.gov/xlibrary/assets/dhs-risk-lexicon-2010.pdf.

DHS. 2021. "Domestic Nuclear Detection Office." https://www.dhs.gov/domestic-nuclear-detection-office.

Director of Central Intelligence. 1986. *The Likelihood of Nuclear Acts by Terrorist Groups.* Langley, VA: Central Intelligence Agency.

DOE (Department of Energy). 2015. "Nuclear Explosive and Weapon Surety Program." DOE Order 452.1E. www.directives.doe.gov.

Dolan, P.E., ed. 1972. "Capabilities of Nuclear Weapons." In *Defense Nuclear Agency Effects Manual 1.* July 1. Washington, DC: Defense Nuclear Agency.

DOS (U.S. Department of State). 1966. *Crisis Over Berlin, American Policy Concerning the Soviet Threats to Berlin: November 1958–December 1962*, Part 1. Historical Studies Division (Research Project 614-A). Washington, DC: U.S. Department of State.

DOS. 2009. *The Global Initiative to Combat Nuclear Terrorism.* https://2009-2017.state.gov/t/isn/c18406.htm.

Downes, R.J., and C. Hobbs. 2017. "Nuclear Terrorism and Virtual Risk: Implications for Prediction and the Utility of Models." *European Journal of International Security* 2(2):203–222. https://doi.org/10.1017/eis.2017.5.

Dresch, F.W., and S. Baum. 1973. *Analysis of the US and USSR Potential for Economic Recovery Following a Nuclear Attack.* Menlo Park, CA: Stanford Strategic Studies Center.

Dresher, M. 1951. *Theory and Applications of Games of Strategy.* Santa Monica, CA: RAND Corporation.

Dunn, L.A. 2005. *Can al Qaeda Be Deterred from Using Nuclear Weapons?* Occasional Paper 3. Center for the Study of Weapons of Mass Destruction. Washington, DC: National Defense University Press.

Earnhardt, R.L., B. Hyatt, and N. Roth. 2021. "A Threat to Confront: Far-Right Extremists and Nuclear Terrorism." *Bulletin of the Atomic Scientists.* January 14. https://thebulletin.org/2021/01/a-threat-to-confront-far-right-extremists-and-nuclear-terrorism.

Eden, L. 2006. *Whole World on Fire: Organizations, Knowledge, and Nuclear Weapons Devastation.* Ithaca, NY: Cornell University Press.

Edwards, W. 1953. "Probability-Preferences in Gambling." *The American Journal of Psychology* 66(3):349–364.

Edwards, W. 1954. "Probability-Preferences Among Bets with Differing Expected Values." *The American Journal of Psychology* 67(1):56–67.

Eisenbud, M., and T.F. Gesell. 1997. *Environmental Radioactivity from Natural, Industrial and Military Sources: From Natural, Industrial and Military Sources*, 4th ed. San Diego: Academic Press.

Ellsberg, D. 2017. *The Doomsday Machine: Confessions of a Nuclear War Planner.* New York: Bloomsbury.

Emery, J.R. 2021. "Moral Choices Without Moral Language: 1950s Political-Military Wargaming at the RAND Corporation." *Texas National Security Review* 4(4):11–31.

Epstein, S. 1994. "Integration of the Cognitive and the Psychodynamic Unconscious." *American Psychologist* 49(8):709.

Etchegary, H., J.E.C. Lee, L. Lemyre, and D. Krewski. 2008. "Canada's Representation of Chemical, Biological, Radiological, Nuclear, and Explosive (CBRNE) Terrorism: A Content Analysis." *Human and Ecological Risk Assessment* 14(3):479.

Ezell, C.E., S.P. Bennett, D. von Winterfeldt, J. Sokolowski, and A.J. Collins. 2010. "Probabilistic Risk Analysis and Terrorism Risk." *Risk Analysis* 30(4):575–590.

Faculty of Societal Safety Sciences. 2018. *The Fukushima and Tohoku Disaster: A Review of the Five-Year Reconstruction Efforts*. Kansai University. Cambridge, MA: Butterworth-Heinemann.

Ferguson, C.D., W.C. Potter, and A. Sands. 2005. *The Four Faces of Nuclear Terrorism*. Abingdon, UK: Routledge.

Ferrer, R.A., A. Maclay, P.M. Litvak, and J.S. Lerner. 2017. "Revisiting the Effects of Anger on Risk-Taking: Empirical and Meta-Analytic Evidence for Differences Between Males and Females." *Journal of Behavioral Decision Making* 30(2):516–526. https://doi.org/10.1002/bdm.1971.

Finocchiaro, M.A. 1994. "Two Empirical Approaches to the Study of Reasoning." *Informal Logic* 16(1).

Fischer, K., and H. Jungermann. 1996. "Rarely Occurring Headaches and Rarely Occurring Blindness: Is Rarely = Rarely? The Meaning of Verbal Frequentistic Labels in Specific Medical Contexts." *Journal of Behavioral Decision Making* 9(3):153–172.

Fischhoff, B., P. Slovic, and S. Lichtenstein. 1978. "Fault Trees: Sensitivity of Estimated Failure Probabilities to Problem Representation." *Journal of Experimental Psychology: Human Perception and Performance* 4(2):330–344. https://doi.org/10.1037/0096-1523.4.2.330.

Flynn, J., and P. Slovic. 1993. "Nuclear Wastes and Public Trust." *Forum for Applied Research and Public Policy* 8(1):92–101.

Frankel, M., J. Scouras, and G. Ullrich. 2015. *The Uncertain Consequences of Nuclear Weapons Use*. Laurel, MD: Johns Hopkins University Applied Physics Laboratory.

Frankel, M., J. Scouras, and G. Ullrich. 2016. *The New Triad*. Laurel, MD: Johns Hopkins University Applied Physics Laboratory.

Freedman, L. 2003. *The Evolution of Nuclear Strategy*, 3rd ed. New York: Palgrave Macmillan.

Freeman, C.R. 2010. *Bayesian Network Analysis of Nuclear Acquisitions*. Master's thesis, Texas A&M University.

Friedman, J.A., J.S. Lerner, and R. Zeckhauser. 2017. "Behavioral Consequences of Probabilistic Precision: Experimental Evidence from National Security Professionals." *International Organization* 71(4):803–826.

Gaertner, J.P., and G.A. Teagarden. 2006. "Development, Application, and Implementation of RAMCAP to Characterize Nuclear Power Plant Risk from Terrorism." *Proceedings of the International Conference on Nuclear Engineering*. https://www.osti.gov/biblio/20995670-development-application-implementation-ramcap-characterize-nuclear-power-plant-risk-from-terrorism.

Gaidow, S. 2007. "Quest for Credibility: Australian Defence Risk Management Framework." *Defense and Security Analysis* 23(4):379–387. https://doi.org/10.1080/14751790701752428.

GAO (Government Accountability Office). 2004a. *DOE Must Address Significant Issues to Meet the Requirements of the New Design Basis Threat*. Subcommittee on National Security, Emerging Threats, and International Relations, Committee on Government Reform, U.S. House of Representatives. Washington, DC: Government Accountability Office.

GAO. 2004b. *Nuclear Regulation: NRC Needs to More Aggressively and Comprehensively Resolve Issues Related to the Davis-Besse Nuclear Power Plant's Shutdown*. Washington, DC: Government Accountability Office.

GAO. 2014. *Nuclear Security: NNSA Should Establish a Clear Vision and Path Forward for Its Security Program*. Washington, DC: Government Accountability Office. https://www.gao.gov/products/gao-14-208.

Garrick, B.J. 2008. *Quantifying and Controlling Catastrophic Risks*. Cambridge, MA: Academic Press.

Gartenstein-Ross, D., M. Shear, and D. Jones. 2019. *Virtual Plotters. Drones. Weaponized AI?: Violent Non-state Actors as Deadly Early Adopter*. Valens Global. https://valensglobal.com/virtual-plotters-drones-weaponized-ai-violent-non-state-actors-as-deadly-early-adopters.

Gerasimov, V. 2016. "The Value of Science Is in the Foresight: New Challenges Demand Rethinking the Forms and Methods of Carrying Out Combat Operations." *Military Review* 96(1):23.

Giesecke, J.A., W.J. Burns, A. Barrett, E. Bayrak, A. Rose, P. Slovic, and M. Suher. 2012. "Assessment of the Regional Economic Impacts of Catastrophic Events: CGE Analysis of Resource Loss and Behavioral Effects of an RDD Attack Scenario." *Risk Analysis: An International Journal* 32(4):583–600.

Glasstone, S., and P.J. Dolan. 1977. *The Effects of Nuclear Weapons*, 3rd ed. Technical Report. OSTI Identifier 6852629. Washington, DC: Department of Defense. https://doi.org/10.2172/6852629.

Gretter, D.M., and C.R. Plott. 1979. "Economic Theory of Choice and the Preference Reversal Phenomenon." *The American Economic Review* 69(4):623–638.

Hafemeister, D. 2014. "Primer on Nuclear Exchange Models." *AIP Conference Proceedings* 1596(1). https://doi.org/10.1063/1.4876435.
Haywood, Jr., O.G. 1954. "Military Decision and Game Theory." *Journal of the Operations Research Society of America* 2(4):365–385.
Heard, D. 2014. *Statistical Inference Utilizing Agent Based Models*. PhD dissertation. Department of Statistical Science, Duke University.
Helfand, I., L. Forrow, and J. Tiwari. 2002. "Nuclear Terrorism." *British Medical Journal* 324(7333):356–358.
Hellman, M.E. 2011. "How Risky Is Nuclear Optimism?" *Bulletin of the Atomic Scientists* 67(2):47–56.
Hirsch, D., S. Murphy, and B. Ramberg. 1986. "Protecting Reactors from Terrorists." *Bulletin of the Atomic Scientists* 42(3):22–25.
Hirst, C. 2007. "The Paradigm Shift: 11 September and Australia's Strategic Reformation." *Australian Journal of International Affairs* 61(2):175–192. https://doi.org/10.1080/10357710701358345.
Holgate, L.S.H. 2018. "The Enduring Challenge of Nuclear Security Coordination." *Arms Control Today* 48(1):14–19.
Hora, S.C. 2007. "Eliciting Probabilities from Experts." Pp. 129–153 in *Advances in Decision Analysis: From Foundations to Applications*. New York: Cambridge University Press.
Houghton, S.M., M. Simon, K. Aquino, and C.B. Goldberg. 2000. "No Safety in Numbers: Persistence of Biases and Their Effects on Team Risk Perception and Team Decision Making." *Group and Organization Management* 25(4):325–353.
Hruby, J., and M.N. Miller. 2021. *Assessing and Managing the Benefits and Risks of Artificial Intelligence in Nuclear-Weapon Systems*. Nuclear Threat Initiative. https://www.nti.org/analysis/articles/assessing-and-managing-the-benefits-and-risks-of-artificial-intelligence-in-nuclear-weapon-systems.
Hughes, P., and E. White. 2010. "The Space Shuttle *Challenger* Disaster: A Classic Example of Groupthink." *Ethics and Critical Thinking Journal* 2010(3).
Ice, L., J. Scouras, K. Rooker, R. Leonard, and D. McGarvey. 2019. *Game Theory and Nuclear Stability in Northeast Asia*. Laurel, MD: Johns Hopkins University Applied Physics Laboratory.
Iklé, F.C. 1958. *The Social Impact of Bomb Destruction*. Norman: University of Oklahoma Press.
IOM (Institute of Medicine). 1986. *The Medical Implications of Nuclear War*. Washington, DC: National Academy Press.
ISO (International Organization for Standardization). 2018. *Risk Management: Guidelines*. https://www.iso.org/obp/ui/#iso:std:iso:31000:ed-2:v1:en.
JAEIC (Joint Atomic Energy Intelligence Committee). 1976. *The Likelihood of the Acquisition of Nuclear Weapons by Foreign Terrorist Groups for Use Against the United States*. Washington, DC: U.S. Intelligence Board.
Jasanoff, S. 1986. "Risk Management and Political Culture: A Comparative Study of Science in the Policy Context." In *Social Research Perspectives: Occasional Reports on Current Topics*. New York: Russell Sage Foundation.
Jenkins, B.M. 2008. *Will Terrorists Go Nuclear?* New York: Prometheus Publications.
Jervis, R. 1988. "The Political Effects of Nuclear Weapons." *International Security* 13(2):80–90.
Johnson, B.B., and P. Slovic. 1995. "Presenting Uncertainty in Health Risk Assessment: Initial Studies of Its Effects on Risk Perception and Trust." *Risk Analysis* 15(4):485–494.
Johnston, J.H., J.A. Cannon-Bowers, and E. Salas. 1998. "Tactical Decision Making Under Stress (TADMUS): Mapping a Program of Research to a Real World Incident—The *USS Vincennes*." Paper presented at RTO HFM Symposium on Collaborative Crew Performance in Complex Operational Systems. April 20–22. Edinburg, UK.
JSOU (Joint Special Operations University) Strategic Studies Department. 2013. *Special Operations Forces Interagency Counterterrorism Reference Manual*, 3rd ed. MacDill Air Force Base, FL: JSOU Press.
Kadane, J.B., and L.J. Wolfson. 1998. "Experiences in Elicitation." *Statistician* 47(1):3–19.
Kahan, D.M., D. Braman, G.L. Cohen, J. Gastil, and P. Slovic. 2010. "Who Fears the HPV Vaccine, Who Doesn't, and Why? An Experimental Study of the Mechanisms of Cultural Cognition." *Law and Human Behavior* 34(6):501–516.
Kahneman, D. 2002. "Maps of Bounded Rationality: A Perspective on Intuitive Judgment and Choice." *Nobel Prize Lecture* 8(1):351–401.
Kahneman, D. 2011. *Thinking, Fast and Slow*. New York: Farrar, Straus and Giroux.

Kahneman, D., P. Slovic, and A. Tversky. 1982. *Judgment Under Uncertainty: Heuristics and Biases*. Cambridge, UK: Cambridge University Press.

Kaner, S. 2014. *Facilitator's Guide to Participatory Decision-Making*. San Francisco, CA: Jossey-Bass.

Kaplan, S., and B.J. Garrick. 1981. "On the Quantitative Definition of Risk." *Risk Analysis* 1(1):11–27.

Karamoskos, P. 2009. "Nuclear Terrorism and Nuclear Medicine—Removing Weapons Grade Uranium from the Nuclear Supply Chain." *ANZ Nuclear Medicine* 40(2):8–15.

Kasperson, R.E., O. Renn, P. Slovic, H.S. Brown, J. Emel, R. Goble, J.X. Kasperson, and S. Ratick. 1988. "The Social Amplification of Risk: A Conceptual Framework." *Risk Analysis* 8(2).

Katz, A., and S.R. Osdoby. 1982. *The Social and Economic Effects of Nuclear War*. Policy Analysis No. 9. April 21. CATO Institute. https://www.cato.org/policy-analysis/social-economic-effects-nuclear-war.

Keeney, R.L., and H. Raiffa, 1976. *Decisions with Multiple Objectives: Preferences and Value Trade-Offs*. Cambridge, UK: Cambridge University Press.

Kennedy, R.F. 1999. *Thirteen Days: A Memoir of the Cuban Missile Crisis*. New York: W.W. Norton and Company.

Kobe, D.H. 1962. "A Theory of Catalytic War." *Journal of Conflict Resolution* 6(2):125–142.

Korda, M., and H. Kristensen. 2021. "China Is Building a Second Nuclear Missile Silo Field." *Strategic Security* (blog). July 26. Federation of American Scientists. https://fas.org/blogs/security/2021/07/china-is-building-a-second-nuclear-missile-silo-field.

Kucik, P., and E. Paté-Cornell. 2012. "Counterinsurgency: A Utility-Based Analysis of Different Strategies." *Military Operations Research* 17(4):5–23. https://doi.org/10.5711/1082598317405.

Kumar, R.S.S., D.O. Brien, K. Albert, S. Viljöen, and J. Snover. 2019. "Failure Modes in Machine Learning Systems." *arXiv*. https://doi.org/10.48550/arXiv.1911.11034.

Lambiase, M.J., L.D. Kubzansky, and R.C. Thurston. 2014. "Prospective Study of Anxiety and Incident Stroke." *Stroke* 45:438–443. https://doi.org/10.1161/STROKEAHA.113.003741.

Larson, E.V. 2019. "Force Planning Scenarios, 1945–2016: Their Origins and Use in Defense Strategic Planning." Santa Monica, CA: RAND Arroyo Center.

Lerner, J.S., and D. Keltner. 2001. "Fear, Anger, and Risk." *Journal of Personality and Social Psychology* 81(1):146–159. https://doi.org/10.1037/0022-3514.81.1.146.

Lerner, J.S., and P.E. Tetlock. 1999. "Accounting for the Effects of Accountability." *Psychological Bulletin* 125(2):255–275. https://doi.org/10.1037/0033-2909.125.2.255.

Lerner, J.S., R.M. Gonzalez, D.A. Small, and B. Fischoff. 2003. "Effects of Fear and Anger on Perceived Risks of Terrorism: A National Field Experiment." *Psychological Science* 14(2):144–150. https://doi.org/10.1111/1467-9280.01433.

Lerner, J.S., L. Yi, P. Valdesolo, and K.S. Kassam. 2015. "Emotion and Decision Making." *Annual Review of Psychology* 66:799–823. https://doi.org/10.1146/annurev-psych-010213-115043.

Leventhal, P., and Y. Alexander. 1987. *Preventing Nuclear Terrorism: The Report and Papers of the International Task Force on Prevention of Nuclear Terrorism*. Lanham, MD: Lexington Books.

Lewis, J. 2018. *The 2020 Commission Report on the North Korean Nuclear Attacks Against the United States*. Boston, MA: Houghton Mifflin Harcourt.

Lichtenstein, S., and B. Fischhoff. 1980. "Training for Calibration." *Organizational Behavior and Human Performance* 26(2):149–171.

Lichtenstein, S., and P. Slovic. 2006. *The Construction of Preference*. Cambridge, UK: Cambridge University Press.

Lichtenstein, S., P. Slovic, B. Fischhoff, M. Layman, and B. Combs. 1978. "Judged Frequency of Lethal Events." *Journal of Experimental Psychology: Human Learning and Memory* 4(6):551–578. https://doi.org/10.1037/0278-7393.4.6.551.

Lieber, K.A., and D.G. Press. 2013. "Why States Won't Give Nuclear Weapons to Terrorists." *International Security* 38(1):80.

Lifton, R.J. 1967. *Death in Life: Survivors of Hiroshima*. New York: Random House.

Lin, S.-W., and V.M. Bier. 2008. "A Study of Expert Overconfidence." *Reliability Engineering and System Safety* 93(5):711–721.

Loewenstein, G.F., W.E.U. Weber, C.K. Hsee, and E.S. Welch. 2001. "Risk as Feelings." *Psychological Bulletin* 127(2):267–286.

Løvold, M., B. Fihn, and T. Nash. 2013. "Humanitarian Perspectives and the Campaign for an International Ban on Weapons." Pp. 145–155 in *Viewing Nuclear Weapons Through a Humanitarian Lens*, J. Borrie and T. Caughley, eds. Geneva: United Nations Institute for Disarmament Research.

Lumb, R.F., F.P. Cotter, G. Charnoff, P. Grady, A.J. O'Donnell, Jr., L.H. Roddis, and F.H. Tingey. 1967. *Report to the Atomic Energy Commission by the Ad Hoc Advisory Panel on Safeguarding Special Nuclear Material.* Washington, DC: Atomic Energy Commission.

Lüth, V.G. 2013. "Wolfgang K.H. Panofsky: Scientist and Arms-Control Expert." *Annual Review of Nuclear and Particle Science* 63(1):1–20.

Lynn, L.E. 1969. "The SIOP." Memorandum from Laurence Lynn, Jr. to Dr. Kissinger, p. 2. November 8. Declassified E.O. 12958, Sect. 3.6, 2004. Mandatory Review Release to the National Security Archive. http://www2.gwu.edu/~nsarchiv/NSAEBB/NSAEBB173/SIOP-3.pdf.

Makridis, C., and J.T. Rothwell. 2020. "The Real Cost of Political Polarization: Evidence from the COVID-19 Pandemic." *VoxEU* (blog). July 10. Center for Economic Policy Research. https://voxeu.org/article/real-cost-political-polarisation.

McGuire, R.K. 2008. "Probabilistic Seismic Hazard Analysis: Early History." *Earthquake Engineering and Structural Dynamics* 37(3):329–338.

McInnis, K.J., and J.W. Rollins. 2018. *The National Security Council: Background and Issues for Congress.* Congressional Research Service. https://purl.fdlp.gov/GPO/gpo136868.

McIntosh, C., and I. Storey. 2018. "Between Acquisition and Use: Assessing the Likelihood of Nuclear Terrorism." *International Studies Quarterly* 62(2):289–300.

McKinley, E. 2021. "The Superforecasters." *DailyFX*. November 15. https://www.dailyfx.com/forex/fundamental/article/special_report/2021/11/15/The-Superforecasters.html.

McNeil, B.J., S.G. Pauker, H.C. Sox, Jr., and A. Tversky. 1982. "On the Elicitation of Preferences for Alternative Therapies." *New England Journal of Medicine* 306(21):1259–1262.

Mellers, B., L. Ungar, J. Baron, J. Ramos, B. Gurcay, K. Fincher, S.E. Scott, D. Moore, P. Atanasov, and S.A. Swift. 2014. "Psychological Strategies for Winning a Geopolitical Forecasting Tournament." *Psychological Science* 25(5):1106–1115.

Merrick, J., and G. Parnell. 2011. "A Comparative Analysis of PRA and Intelligent Adversary Methods for Counterterrorism Risk Management." *Risk Analysis* 31(9):1488–1510.

Moakler, M.W. 2015. "The VNTK System." *Countering WMD Journal* Fall/Winter(13):6–10.

Moniz, E.J., and S. Nunn. 2019. "The Return of Doomsday: The New Nuclear Arms Race—and How Washington and Moscow Can Stop It." *Foreign Affairs* September/October:150–161.

Moore, D.A. 2020. "Perfectly Confident: How to Calibrate Your Decisions Wisely." *Harper Business* May 26.

Moore, D.A., and P.J. Healy. 2008. "The Trouble with Overconfidence." *Psychological Review* 115(2):502–517. https://doi.org/10.1037/0033-295X.115.2.502.

Morewedge, A.K., H. Yoon, I. Scopelliti, C.W. Symborski, J.H. Korris, and K.S. Kassam. 2015. "Debiasing Decisions: Improved Decision Making with a Single Training Intervention." *Policy Insights from the Behavioral and Brain Sciences* 2(1):129–140. https://doi.org/10.1177/2372732215600886.

Morgan, G.P., M.J. Lanham, W. Frankenstein, and K.M. Carley. 2017. "Sociocultural Models of Nuclear Deterrence." *IEEE Transactions on Computational Social Systems* 4(3):121–134.

Morgan, M.G., B. Fischoff, A. Bostrom, and C.J. Atman. 2002. *Risk Communications: A Mental Models Approach.* Cambridge, UK: Cambridge University Press.

Mowatt-Larssen, R., and G.T. Allison. 2010. *Al Qaeda Weapons of Mass Destruction Threat: Hype or Reality?* Boston, MA: Belfer Center for Science and International Affairs.

Murphy, D.M., and M.E. Paté-Cornell. 1996. "The SAM Framework: A Systems Analysis Approach to Modeling the Effects of Management on Human Behavior in Risk Analysis." *Risk Analysis* 16(4):501–515.

Murphy, H.L., J.R. Rempel, and J.E. Beck. 1975. *Slanting in New Basements for Combined Nuclear Weapons Effects: A Consolidated Printing of Four Technical Reports. Volumes 1, 2 and 3. Final Report.* Menlo Park, CA: Stanford Research Institute.

Nagel, K., R.J. Beckman, and C.L. Barrett. 1999. *TRANSIMS for Urban Planning.* Sixth International Conference on Computers in Urban Planning and Urban Management. Venice, Italy.

Narang, V. 2010. "Posturing for Peace? Pakistan's Nuclear Postures and South Asian Stability." *International Security* 34(3):38. https://doi.org/http://dx.doi.org/10.1162/isec.2010.34.3.38.

NAS (National Academy of Sciences). 2015. *Brazil-U.S. Workshop on Strengthening the Culture of Nuclear Safety and Security: Summary of a Workshop*. Washington, DC: The National Academies Press.

NASEM (National Academies of Sciences, Engineering, and Medicine). 2016. *Lessons Learned from the Fukushima Nuclear Accident for Improving Safety and Security of U.S. Nuclear Plants: Phase 2*. Washington, DC: The National Academies Press.

Nasstrom, J.S., G. Sugiyama, R.L. Baskett, S.C. Larsen, and M.M. Bradley. 2007. "The National Atmospheric Release Advisory Center Modelling and Decision-Making System for Radiological and Nuclear Emergency Preparedness and Response." *International Journal of Emergency Management* 4(3):524–550.

National Research Council. 1996. *Understanding Risk: Informing Decisions in a Democratic Society*. Washington, DC: National Academy Press.

National Research Council. 1999. *Protecting Nuclear Weapons Material in Russia*. Washington, DC: National Academy Press.

National Research Council. 2002. *Making the Nation Safer: The Role of Science and Technology in Countering Terrorism*. Washington, DC: The National Academies Press.

National Research Council. 2006. *Safety and Security of Commercial Spent Nuclear Fuel Storage: Public Report*. Washington, DC: The National Academies Press.

National Research Council. 2008. *Department of Homeland Security Bioterrorism Risk Assessment: A Call for Change*. Washington, DC: The National Academies Press.

National Research Council. 2009. *Global Security Engagement: A New Model for Cooperative Threat Reduction*. Washington, DC: The National Academies Press.

National Research Council. 2011. *Understanding and Managing Risk in Security Systems for the DOE Nuclear Weapons Complex (Abbreviated Version)*. Washington, DC: The National Academies Press.

National Research Council. 2013. *Improving the Assessment of the Proliferation Risk of Nuclear Fuel Cycles*. Washington, DC: The National Academies Press.

NRC (U.S. Nuclear Regulatory Commission). 1975. *Reactor Safety Study: An Assessment of Accident Risks in U.S. Commercial Nuclear Power Plants*. WASH-1400. Washington, DC.

NRC. 1990. *Severe Accident Risks: An Assessment for Five U.S. Nuclear Power Plants—Final Summary Report*. Division of Systems Research, Office of Nuclear Regulatory Research. Washington, DC.

NRC. 2019. "Backgrounder on Force-on-Force Security Inspections." https://www.nrc.gov/reading-rm/doc-collections/fact-sheets/force-on-force-bg.html.

NTI (Nuclear Threat Initiative). 2002. "10 Plus 10 Over 10 Program." https://www.nti.org/education-center/treaties-and-regimes/global-partnership-against-spread-weapons-and-materials-mass-destruction-10-plus-10-over-10-program.

Obama, B. 2009. "Organization of the National Security Council System." In *Presidential Policy Directive-1*. Washington, DC: The White House.

ODNI (Office of the Director of National Intelligence). 2021. *Annual Threat Assessment of the U.S. Intelligence Community*. Washington, DC. https://www.dni.gov/files/ODNI/documents/assessments/ATA-2021-Unclassified-Report.pdf.

Office of the Coordinator for Counterterrorism. 2012. "Strategic Assessment." In *Country Reports on Terrorism 2011*. Washington, DC: U.S. Department of State. https://2009-2017.state.gov/j/ct/rls/crt/2011/195540.htm.

O'Hagan, A., C.E. Buck, A. Daneshkhah, J.R. Eiser, P.H. Garthwaite, D.J. Jenkinson, J.E. Oakley, and T. Rakow. 2006. *Uncertain Judgements: Eliciting Experts' Probabilities*. West Sussex, UK: John Wiley and Sons, Ltd.

O'Neill, B. 1994. "Game Theory Models of Peace and War." Pp. 995–1053 in *Handbook of Game Theory with Economic Applications*, R. Aumann and S. Hart, eds. Vol. 2 of *Handbooks in Economics*, K. Arrow and M. Intriligator, eds. Amsterdam: Elsevier.

OSD (Office of the Secretary of Defense). 2010. *Nuclear Posture Review*. Washington, DC. https://dod.defense.gov/Portals/1/features/defenseReviews/NPR/2010_Nuclear_Posture_Review_Report.pdf.

OSD. 2018. *Nuclear Posture Review*. Washington, DC. https://media.defense.gov/2018/Feb/02/2001872886/-1/-1/1/2018-NUCLEAR-POSTURE-REVIEW-FINAL-REPORT.PDF.

OSD. 2019. *Missile Defense Review*. https://www.defense.gov/Portals/1/Interactive/2018/11-2019-Missile-Defense-Review/The%202019%20MDR_Executive%20Summary.pdf.

OTA (Office of Technology Assessment). 1979. *The Effects of Nuclear War*. Washington, DC: U.S. Government Printing Office.

Ouagrham-Gormley, S.B. 2007. "Nuclear Terrorist's Fatal Assumptions." *Bulletin of the Atomic Scientists* 22.

Parikh, N., S. Swarup, P.E. Stretz, C.M. Rivers, B.L. Lewis, M.V. Marathe, S.G. Eubank, C.L. Barrett, K. Lum, and Y. Chungbaek. 2013. "Modeling Human Behavior in the Aftermath of a Hypothetical Improvised Nuclear Detonation." Pp. 949–956 in *12th International Conference on Autonomous Agents and Multiagent Systems.*

Parnell, G.S., G.M. Smith, and F.I. Moxley. 2011. "Intelligent Adversary Risk Analysis: A Bioterrorism Risk Management Model." *Risk Analysis* 30:32–48.

Paté-Cornell, M.E. 1984. "Fault Trees vs. Event Trees in Reliability Analysis." *Risk Analysis* 4(3):177–186.

Paté-Cornell, M.E. 1986. "Warning Systems in Risk Management." *Risk Analysis* 6(2):223–234.

Paté-Cornell, M.E. 1996. "Uncertainties in Risk Analysis: Six Levels of Treatment." *Reliability Engineering and System Safety* 54(2):95–111. https://doi.org/10.1016/S0951-8320(96)00067-1.

Paté-Cornell, M.E. 2009. "Risks and Games: Intelligent Actors and Fallible Systems." In *Proceedings of the Second International Symposium on Engineering Systems.* Cambridge, MA: Massachusetts Institute of Technology.

Paté-Cornell, M.E. 2011. "An Introduction to Probabilistic Risk Analysis for Engineered Systems." In *Wiley Encyclopedia of Operations Research and Management Science*, J.J. Cochran, L.A. Cox, P. Keskinocak, J.P. Kharoufeh, and J.C. Smith, eds. https://doi.org/10.1002/9780470400531.eorms0680.

Paté-Cornell, M.E., and P.S. Fischbeck. 1994. "Risk Management for the Tiles of the Space Shuttle." *Interfaces* 24(1):64–86.

Paté-Cornell, M.E., and S. Guikema. 2002. "Probabilistic Modeling of Terrorist Threats: A Systems Analysis Approach to Setting Priorities Among Countermeasures." *Military Operations Research* 7(4):5–23.

Paté-Cornell, M.E., and J.E. Neu. 1985. "Warning Systems and Defense Policy: A Reliability Model for the Command and Control of US Nuclear Forces." *Risk Analysis* 5(2):121–138.

Perera, R. 2005. *International Convention for the Suppression of Acts of Nuclear Terrorism.* New York: United Nations Audiovisual Library of International Law. https://legal.un.org/avl/ha/icsant/icsant.html.

Perrow, C. 2011. *Normal Accidents.* Princeton, NJ: Princeton University Press.

Peters, E. 2020. *Innumeracy in the Wild: Misunderstanding and Misusing Numbers.* New York: Oxford University Press.

Phelps, E.A, K.M. Lempert, and P. Sokol-Hessner. 2014. "Emotion and Decision Making: Multiple Modulatory Neural Circuits." *Annual Review of Neuroscience* 37:262–387. https://doi.org/10.1146/annurev-neuro-071013-014119.

Pidgeon, N., R.E. Kasperson, and P. Slovic. 2003. *The Social Amplification of Risk.* Cambridge, UK: Cambridge University Press.

Plous, S. 1993. *The Psychology of Judgment and Decision Making.* New York: McGraw-Hill Book Company.

Purvis, J.W. 1999. *Sabotage at Nuclear Power Plants.* Albuquerque, NM: Sandia National Laboratories.

Quinlan, M. 2009. *Thinking About Nuclear Weapons: Principles, Problems, Prospects.* New York: Oxford University Press.

Rajivan, P., and N.J. Cooke. 2018. "Information-Pooling Bias in Collaborative Security Incident Correlation Analysis." *Human Factors* 60(5):626–639.

Ramberg, B. 1985. *Nuclear Power Plants as Weapons for the Enemy: An Unrecognized Military Peril.* Berkeley: University of California Press.

Rampton, R. 2011. "Fukushima Disaster Not 'Unforeseen'—NRC Commissioner." *Reuters: Regulatory News* August 3. https://www.reuters.com/article/usa-nuclear-apostolakis/fukushima-disaster-not-unforeseen-nrc-commissioner-idINN1E77211Y20110803.

RAND Corporation. 1956. *Protecting U.S. Power to Strike Back in the 1950s and 1960s.* Santa Monica, CA.

Rausand, M., and A. Hoyland. 2003. *System Reliability Theory: Models, Statistical Methods, and Applications*, 2nd ed. In *Wiley Series in Probability and Statistics.* Hoboken, NJ: Wiley Interscience.

Richelson, J.T. 2009. *Defusing Armageddon: Inside NEST, America's Secret Nuclear Bomb Squad.* New York: W.W. Norton and Company.

Rios Insua, D., J. Rios, and D. Banks. 2012. "Adversarial Risk Analysis." *Journal of the American Statistical Association* 104(486):841–854. https://doi.org/10.1198/jasa.2009.0155.

Roberts, B. 2021. *Emerging and Disruptive Technologies, Multi-Domain Complexity, and Strategic Stability: A Review and Assessment of the Literature.* Livermore, CA: Lawrence Livermore National Laboratory.

Rosoff, H., and von Winterfeldt, D. 2007. "A Risk and Economic Analysis of Dirty Bomb Attacks on the Port of Los Angeles and Long Beach." *Risk Analysis* 27(3):533–546.

Rottenstreich, Y., and C.K. Hsee. 2001. "Money, Kisses, and Electric Shocks: On the Affective Psychology of Risk." *Psychological Science* 12(3):185–190.

Rowe, G., and G. Wright. 1999. "The Delphi Technique as a Forecasting Tool: Issues and Analysis." *International Journal of Forecasting* 15(4):353–375.

Sagan, S.D. 1987. "SIOP-62: The Nuclear War Plan Briefing to President Kennedy." *International Security* 12(1):22–51.

Sagan, S.D. 1993. *The Limits of Safety: Organizations, Accidents, and Nuclear Weapons.* Princeton, NJ: Princeton University Press.

Sagan, S.D. 2000. "The Commitment Trap." *International Security* 24(4):85–115.

Sagan, S.D. 2018. "Armed and Dangerous: When Dictators Get the Bomb." *Foreign Affairs.* https://www.foreignaffairs.com/articles/north-korea/2018-10-15/armed-and-dangerous.

Salter, C.A. 2001. "Psychological Effects of Nuclear and Radiological Warfare." *Military Medicine* 166(Suppl 2):17–18. https://doi.org/10.1093/milmed/166.suppl_2.17.

Sandoz, J.F. 2001. *Red Teaming: A Means to Military Transformation.* Joint Advanced Warfighting Program. Alexandria, VA: Institute for Defense Analyses. https://apps.dtic.mil/sti/pdfs/ADA388176.pdf.

Savage, L.J. 1954. *The Foundations of Statistics.* Hoboken, NJ: John Wiley and Sons.

Schelling, T.C. 1958. *The Reciprocal Fear of Surprise Attack.* Santa Monica, CA: RAND Corporation.

Schelling, T.C. 1960. "The Threat That Leaves Something to Chance." Pp. 187–203 in *The Strategy of Conflict.* Cambridge, MA: Harvard University Press.

Schelling, T.C. 1980. *The Strategy of Conflict: With a New Preface by the Author.* Cambridge, MA: Harvard University Press.

Schelling, T.C. 2008. *Arms and Influence.* New Haven, CT: Yale University Press.

Schmidt, E., B. Work, S. Catz, S. Chien, C. Darby, K. Ford, J.-M. Griffiths, et al. 2021. *Final Report.* National Security Commission on Artificial Intelligence. https://irp.fas.org/offdocs/ai-commission.pdf.

Schwarz, R.M. 2002. *The Skilled Facilitator: A Comprehensive Resource for Consultants, Facilitators, Managers, Trainers, and Coaches.* San Francisco, CA: Jossey-Bass.

Scoblic, J.P., and P.E. Tetlock. 2020. "A Better Crystal Ball: The Right Way to Think About the Future." *Foreign Affairs* 99(6):10–19.

Scouras, J. 2019. "Nuclear War as a Global Catastrophic Risk." *Journal of Benefit-Cost Analysis* 10(2):274–295.

Scouras, J., A. Bennett, J.M. Booker, M.E. Hellman, E.T. Toton, M.J. Frankel, G.W. Ullrich, and D. Boyd. 2021. *On Assessing the Risk of Nuclear War*, J. Scouras, ed. Laurel, MA: Johns Hopkins Applied Physics Laboratory.

Selten, R., and R. Tietz. 1966. "A Formal Theory of Security Equilibria." Pp. 185–202 in *The Future of the International Strategic System*, R.N. Rosecrance, ed. San Francisco, CA: Chandler.

Shahzad, A., K.N. Das, and G.N. Peshimam. 2022. "India Says It Accidentally Fired Missile into Pakistan." *Reuters* March 11.

Shapiro, J.N. 2013. *The Terrorist's Dilemma: Managing Violent Covert Organizations.* Princeton, NJ: Princeton University Press.

Simon, H.A. 1957. *Models of Man: Social and Rational—Mathematical Essays on Rational Human Behavior in a Social Setting.* Hoboken, NJ: Wiley.

Slovic, P. 1987. "Perception of Risk." *Science* 236(4799):280–285.

Slovic, P. 1990. "Perception of Risk from Radiation." In *Radiation Protection Today: The NCRP at Sixty Years.* Pp. 73–97 (No. 11) in *Proceedings of the Twenty-Fifth Annual Meeting of the National Council on Radiation Protection and Measurements*, W.K. Sinclair, ed. Bethesda, MD: NCRP.

Slovic, P. 1995. "The Construction of Preference." *American Psychologist* 50(5):364.

Slovic, P. 1999. "Trust, Emotion, Sex, Politics, and Science: Surveying the Risk-Assessment Battlefield." *Risk Analysis* 19(4):689–701.

Slovic, P., and H. Lin. 2020. "The Caveman and the Bomb in the Digital Age." Pp. 39–62 in *Three Tweets to Midnight: Effects of the Global Information Ecosystem on the Risk of Nuclear Conflict*, H.S. Lin and B. Leohrke, eds. Stanford, CA: Hoover Institution Press.

Slovic, P., J. Monahan, and D.G. MacGregor. 2000. "Violence Risk Assessment and Risk Communication: The Effects of Using Actual Cases, Providing Instruction, and Employing Probability Versus Frequency Formats." *Law and Human Behavior* 24(3):271–296.

Slovic, P., C.K. Mertz, D.M. Markowitz, A. Quist, and D. Västfjäll. 2020. "Virtuous Violence from the War Room to Death Row." *Proceedings of the National Academy of Sciences U.S.A.* 117(34):20474–20482.

Sniezek, J.A. 1992. "Groups Under Uncertainty: An Examination of Confidence in Group Decision Making." *Organizational Behavior and Human Decision Processes* 52(1):124–155.

Sokolovskii, V.D., H.S. Dinerstein, L. Goure, and T.W. Wolfe. 1963. *Soviet Military Strategy: A Translation from the Russian of V.D. Sokolovskii with Analysis and Annotation by H. Dinerstein, L. Gouré, and T. Wolfe.* Santa Monica, CA: RAND Corporation.

Srikrishna, D., A.N. Chari, and T. Tisch. 2005. "Deterrence of Nuclear Terrorism with Mobile Radiation Detectors." *Nonproliferation Review* 12(3):573–614.

Starr, C. 1981. "Risk Criteria for Nuclear Power Plants: A Pragmatic Proposal 1." *Risk Analysis* 1(2):113–120.

Stasser, G., and W. Titus. 1985. "Pooling of Unshared Information in Group Decision Making: Biased Information Sampling During Discussion." *Journal of Personality and Social Psychology* 48(6):1467.

Stockfish, J.A. 1975. *Models, Data, and War: A Critique of the Study of Conventional Forces.* Santa Monica, CA: RAND Corporation.

Streetman, S.S. 2011. *From Calculations to Results to Decisions.* Architecture Directorate, Domestic Nuclear Detection Office. Washington, DC: Department of Homeland Security.

Sunstein, C.R. 2003. "Terrorism and Probability Neglect." *Journal of Risk and Uncertainty* 26(2):121–136.

Sutherland, W.J., and M. Burgman. 2015. "Policy Advice: Use Experts Wisely." *Nature News* 526(7573):317.

Swarup, S., K. Lum, C.L. Barrett, K. Bisset, S.G. Eubank, M.V. Marathe, and P. Stretz. 2013. "A Synthetic Information Approach to Urban-Scale Disaster Modeling." *IEEE 16th International Conference on Computational Science and Engineering.* August 17–21. Lancaster, UK.

Talmadge, C. 2017. "Would China Go Nuclear?: Assessing the Risk of Chinese Nuclear Escalation in a Conventional War with the United States." *International Security* 41(4):50–92.

Tenet, G. 2007. *At the Center of the Storm: My Years at the CIA.* New York: HarperCollins.

Tetlock, P.E., and D. Gardner. 2015. *Superforecasting: The Art and Science of Prediction.* New York: Crown Publishers.

Tetlock, P.E., J.L. Husbands, R. Jervis, P.C. Stern, and C. Tilly, eds. 1989. *Behavior, Society, and Nuclear War*, Vol. 1. New York: Oxford University Press.

Tetlock, P.E., J.L. Husbands, R. Jervis, P.C. Stern, and C. Tilly, eds. 1991. *Behavior, Society, and Nuclear War*, Vol. 2. New York: Oxford University Press.

Tønnessen, T.H. 2017. "Islamic State and Technology—A Literature Review." *Perspectives on Terrorism* 11(6):101–111.

Travers, W.D. 2001. *Scoping Paper for a Comprehensive Review of the NRC's Safeguards and Security Programs in Light of the Terrorist Attacks on September 11, 2001.* Rockville, MD: U.S. Nuclear Regulatory Commission.

Trost, L.C., and V.N. Vargas. 2020. *Economic Impacts of a Radiological Dispersal Device.* Albuquerque, NM: Sandia National Laboratories.

Truman, H.S., and J.S. Lay. 1950. *United States Objectives and Programs for National Security.* National Security Council Report 68. https://digitalarchive.wilsoncenter.org/document/116191.

Trump, D.J. 2017. "Organization of the National Security Council, the Homeland Security Council, and Subcommittees." In *National Security Presidential Memorandum—4.* Washington, DC: The White House.

Turner, M.E., and A.R. Pratkanis. 1998. "Twenty-Five Years of Groupthink Theory and Research: Lessons from the Evaluation of a Theory." *Organizational Behavior and Human Decision Processes* 73(2–3):105–115.

Tversky, A., and D. Kahneman. 1973. "Availability: A Heuristic for Judging Frequency and Probability." *Cognitive Psychology* 5(2):207–232. https://doi.org/10.1016/0010-0285(73)90033-9.

Tversky, A., and D. Kahneman. 1974. "Judgment under Uncertainty: Heuristics and Biases." *Science* 185(4157):1124–1131.

Tversky, A., and D. Kahneman. 1983. "Extensional Versus Intuitive Reasoning: The Conjunction Fallacy in Probability Judgment." *Psychological Review* 90(4):293.

Tversky, A., and D.J. Koehler. 1994. "Support Theory: A Nonextensional Representation of Subjective Probability." *Psychological Review* 101(4):547.

UN (United Nations) Security Council. 2004. *Resolution 1540 (2004).* Office for Disarmament Affairs. Washington, DC: UN Security Council.

U.S. House of Representatives. 2007. *Nuclear Weapons: Annual Assessment of the Safety, Performance, and Reliability of the Nation's Stockpile.* Subcommittee on Strategic Forces and Committee on Armed Services. Washington, DC: U.S. Government Accountability Office. https://www.gao.gov/assets/gao-07-243r.pdf.

U.S. Strategic Bombing Surveys. 1947. *Reports of the United States Strategic Bombing Surveys.*

U.S. Strategic Command. 1995. *Essentials of Post-Cold War Deterrence.* https://www.nukestrat.com/us/stratcom/SAGessentials.pdf.

U.S. Strategic Command. 2020. *Nuclear Planning Guidance.*

Van der Bles, A.M., S. van der Linden, A.L.J. Freeman, J. Mitchell, A.B. Galvao, L. Zaval, and D.J. Spiegelhalter. 2019. "Communicating Uncertainty About Facts, Numbers and Science." *Royal Society Open Science* 6(5):181870.

Van der Bles, A.M., S. van der Linden, A.L.J. Freeman, and D.J. Spiegelhalter. 2020. "The Effects of Communication Uncertainty on Public Trust in Facts and Numbers." *Proceedings of the National Academy of Sciences U.S.A.* 117(14):7672–7683. https://doi.org/10.1073/pnas.1913678117.

Vargas, V. 2020. *Economic Impacts of a Radiological Dispersal Device: Presented to NAS April 2020.* Albuquerque, NM: Sandia National Laboratories.

Vargas, V.N., and M.A. Ehlen. 2013. "REAcct: A Scenario Analysis Tool for Rapidly Estimating Economic Impacts of Major Natural and Man-Made Hazards." *Environmentalist* 33(1):76–88. https://doi.org/10.1007/s10669-012-9430-5.

von Hippel, F.N., and M. Schoeppner. 2017. "Economic Losses from a Fire in a Dense-Packed US Spent Fuel Pool." *Science and Global Security* 25(2):80–92.

Walker, J.S. 2001. "Regulating Against Nuclear Terrorism: The Domestic Safeguards Issue, 1970–1979." *Technology and Culture* 42(1):107–132.

Walker, K., J.S. Evans, and D. MacIntosh. 2001. "Use of Expert Judgment in Exposure Assessment. Part I. Characterization of Personal Exposure to Benzene." *Journal of Exposure Science and Environmental Epidemiology* 11(4):308–322.

West, D.M., and J.R. Allen. 2020. *Turning Point: Policymaking in the Era of Artificial Intelligence.* Washington, DC: Brookings Institution Press.

White House. 2017. *National Security Strategy of the United States.* https://trumpwhitehouse.archives.gov/wp-content/uploads/2017/12/NSS-Final-12-18-2017-0905.pdf.

White House. 2018. *National Strategy for Countering Weapons of Mass Destruction Terrorism.* https://www.hsdl.org/?abstract&did=819382.

White House. 2022. "Vice President Harris Advances National Security Norms in Space," Fact Sheet. April 18. https://www.whitehouse.gov/briefing-room/statements-releases/2022/04/18/fact-sheet-vice-president-harris-advances-national-security-norms-in-space.

Whitehead, D.W., C.S. Potter, and S.L. O'Connor. 2007. *Nuclear Power Plant Security Assessment Technical Manual.* SAND2007-5591. Albuquerque, NM: Sandia National Laboratories.

Willis, H.H., A.R. Morral, T.K. Kelly, and J.J. Melby. 2005. "Estimating Terrorism Risk." MG-388-RC. Santa Monica, CA: RAND Corporation.

Wilson, R., and E.A.C. Crouch. 2001. *Risk-Benefit Analysis*, 2nd ed. Center for Risk Analysis. Cambridge, MA: Harvard University.

WINS (World Institute for Nuclear Security). 2016. *Nuclear Security Culture.* Vienna: World Institute for Nuclear Security.

Wittenbaum, G.M., and G. Stasser. 1996. "Management of Information in Small Groups." Pp. 3–28 in *What's Social About Social Cognition? Research on Socially Shared Cognition in Small Groups.* Thousand Oaks, CA: Sage Publications.

Wohlstetter, A. 1952. *A Little Answer and Some Big Questions for the Target Systems Analysis.* Santa Monica, CA: RAND Corporation.

Wohlstetter, A., and H.S. Rowen. 1952. *Campaign Time Pattern, Sortie Rate, and Base Location.* Santa Monica, CA: RAND Corporation.

Woo, G. 2021. "Introduction and Overview of Structured Expert Judgement." In *Expert Judgement in Risk and Decision Analysis*, A. Hanea, G. Nane, T. Bedford, and S. French, eds. Vol. 293 of *International Series in Operations Research and Management Science*, C. Price, ed. Cham: Springer International Publishing. https://doi.org/10.1007/978-3-030-46474-5_22.

Woolf, A.F. 2008. *US Nuclear Weapons: Changes in Policy and Force Structure.* Congressional Research Service. Washington, DC: Library of Congress.
World Nuclear Association. 2021. "Safety of Nuclear Power Reactors." https://www.world-nuclear.org/information-library/safety-and-security/safety-of-plants/safety-of-nuclear-power-reactors.aspx.
Zaitseva, L., and F. Steinhäusler. 2014. *Nuclear Trafficking Issues in the Black Sea Region.* Paris: EU Non-Proliferation Consortium. https://www.sipri.org/publications/2014/eu-non-proliferation-papers/nuclear-trafficking-issues-black-sea-region.
Zenko, M. 2006. "Intelligence Estimates of Nuclear Terrorism." *Annals of the American Academy of Political and Social Science* 607(1):87–102.
Zenko, M. 2015. *Red Team: How to Succeed by Thinking Like the Enemy.* New York: Basic Books.
Zhuang, J., and V.M. Bier. 2007. "Balancing Terrorism and Natural Disasters—Defensive Strategy with Endogenous Attacker Effort." *Operations Research* 55(5):976–991.

Appendixes

A

U.S. Strategic Assumptions About Nuclear Risks

U.S. government statements on assumptions associated with nuclear risks can be found in an administration's Nuclear Posture Review, National Security Strategy, Strategic Guidance, National Strategy for Countering Weapons of Mass Destruction Terrorism, and other publicly available documents. The committee found it helpful to review these assumptions in the context of risk analysis approaches. While certainly not a comprehensive list, the following official government statements from these publicly available documents do provide background context for the committee's work. It is noted that as of the time of data collection and briefings for Phase I of the report (Appendix D), the current administration had not yet released its Nuclear Posture Review or National Security Strategy.

ASSUMPTIONS ABOUT THE RISKS POSED BY NUCLEAR WEAPONS USE

"There now exists an unprecedented range and mix of threats, including major conventional, chemical, biological, nuclear, space, and cyber threats, and violent nonstate actors. These developments have produced increased uncertainty and risk" (OSD 2018, p. 1).

"The Nuclear Nonproliferation Treaty is a cornerstone of the nuclear nonproliferation regime. It plays a positive role in building consensus for nonproliferation and enhances international efforts to impose costs on those that would pursue nuclear weapons outside the Treaty" (OSD 2018, p. 1).

ASSUMPTIONS ABOUT THE STRATEGIC INTENT OF ADVERSARIES

"Three main sets of challengers—the revisionist powers of China and Russia, the ... states of Iran and North Korea, and transnational threat organizations, particularly jihadist terrorist groups are actively competing against the United States and our allies" (White House 2017, p. 25).

"Russia considers the United States and the North Atlantic Treaty Organization (NATO) to be the principal threats to its contemporary geopolitical ambitions. Russian strategy and doctrine emphasize the potential coercive and military uses of nuclear weapons. It mistakenly assesses that the threat of nuclear escalation or actual first use of nuclear weapons would serve to 'de-escalate' a conflict on terms favorable to Russia" (OSD 2018, p. 8).

"China continues to increase the number, capabilities, and protection of its nuclear forces. While China's declaratory policy and doctrine have not changed, its lack of transparency regarding the scope and scale of its nuclear modernization program raises questions regarding its future intent" (OSD 2018, p. 11).

"The Iranian regime sponsors terrorism around the world. It is developing more capable ballistic missiles and has the potential to resume its work on nuclear weapons that could threaten the United States and our partners" (White House 2017, p. 26).

"North Korea is ruled as a ruthless dictatorship without regard for human dignity. For more than 25 years, it has pursued nuclear weapons and ballistic missiles in defiance of every commitment it has made. Today, these missiles and weapons threaten the United States and our allies" (White House 2017, p. 26).

ASSUMPTIONS ABOUT THE CAPABILITIES OF ADVERSARIES AND INFORMATION AVAILABLE TO THEM

"Russia possesses significant advantages in its nuclear weapons production capacity and in non-strategic nuclear forces over the U.S. and allies. It is also building a large, diverse, and modern set of non-strategic systems that are dual-capable (may be armed with nuclear or conventional weapons)" (OSD 2018, p. 9).

ASSUMPTIONS ABOUT U.S. STRATEGIC GOALS

"The highest U.S. nuclear policy and strategy priority is to deter potential adversaries from nuclear attack of any scale" (OSD 2018, p. 20).

"The United States has extended nuclear deterrence commitments that assure European, Asian, and Pacific allies. The United States will ensure the credibility and effectiveness of those commitments" (OSD 2018, p. 22).

"Today's U.S. missile defenses provide significant protection against potential North Korean or Iranian ballistic missile strikes against the U.S homeland, and will improve as necessary to stay ahead of missile threats from rogue states" (OSD 2019, p. v).

"We will modernize our nuclear enterprise to ensure that we have the scientific, engineering, and manufacturing capabilities necessary to retain an effective and safe nuclear Triad and respond to future national security threats" (Trump 2017, p. 30).

ASSUMPTIONS ABOUT DETERRENCE

"The United States will maintain a portion of its nuclear forces on alert day-to-day, and retain the option of launching those forces promptly. This posture maximizes decision time and preserves the range of U.S. response options. It also makes clear to potential adversaries that they can have no confidence in strategies intended to destroy our nuclear deterrent forces in a surprise first-strike" (OSD 2018, p. 28).

"The United States has never adopted a 'no first use' policy and, given the contemporary threat environment, such a policy is not justified today. It remains the policy of the United States to retain some ambiguity regarding the precise circumstances that might lead to a U.S. nuclear response" (OSD 2018, p. 22).

The threat of using nuclear weapons in response to a "non-nuclear strategic attack" (including chemical, biological, and cyber) can be an effective deterrent (OSD 2018, p. 22).

ASSUMPTIONS ABOUT NUCLEAR TERRORISM

"Nuclear terrorism remains among the most significant threats to the security of the United States, allies, and partners" (OSD 2018, p. 66).

"The most effective way to reduce the risk of nuclear terrorism is to secure nuclear weapons and materials at their sources" (OSD 2018, p. 67).

"Nuclear and radiological terrorism requires materials that even the most sophisticated terrorists have not to date been able to produce. Because these materials must be acquired, whether through theft or illicit purchase, securing them at their source is among the most urgent security requirements of our age" (White House 2018, p. 6).

B

Types of Uncertainty

There are two distinct types of uncertainty that analysts must address and communicate—uncertainty due to lack of knowledge and that due to inherent randomness (Apostolakis 1990).

The clearest example of inherent randomness (referred to as *aleatory* uncertainty, from the Latin *alea* meaning "dice game") can be illustrated by the flip of a coin or the roll of dice. Even if the coin or dice are fair, and fairly tossed, the exact result each time is inherently random, and not reducible by further study. In the context of nuclear war or terrorism, an example of this random uncertainty is the possibility of a false alarm from a detector. Even if a good estimate of the rate of false alarms is known, whether one will occur on a given day is inherently random. That uncertainty cannot be reduced on the spot (and therefore, at that precise time, reflects randomness) but can be addressed later by more testing of the detector.

Systematic uncertainty due to lack of knowledge (referred to as *epistemic* uncertainty, from the Greek *episteme* meaning "knowledge") can, in principle, be refined (increased or reduced, even if not eliminated) through research if the basis for this uncertainty is recognized and better understood. Decision makers rely on the intelligence community to refine systematic, epistemic uncertainty about the goals, motivations, and capabilities of potential attackers. Their examination of the signals may result in either an increase or a decrease of uncertainties, which in either case must be properly communicated to the decision maker. More generally, decision makers rely on the broader research community to refine understanding of systematic uncertainties about natural, human, and engineered processes.

For systematic uncertainty, the sources of uncertainty need to be recognized or at least anticipated in order to be studied and—once understood—potentially adjusted. The intelligence community often requires at least two independent means of characterization of a phenomenon—for example, "dual phenomenology" in documenting an attack. But unless the sources of uncertainty are fully understood, the messages may not be entirely independent, and in that case are still subject to systematic error. Biases, unrecognized assumptions, and cultural perspectives are among the common sources of systematic biases, which include both systematic errors in measurement and lapses due to conceptual uncertainty (i.e., relevant variables are not even being considered, let alone documented). In addition, pressures to reduce uncertainties may lead to catastrophic misinformation.

In practice, of course, both epistemic and aleatory uncertainties typically come into play in a single decision or question, and can both be addressed by Bayesian probability. For example, there may be systematic uncertainty about the rate of false alarms from a particular detection technology, and that uncertainty might be addressed through experimental research, but randomness still exists about the timing of a false alarm, even after research has been done to address the level of epistemic uncertainty. In some cases, aleatory uncertainty cannot be reduced; for example, one cannot change dice (unless by cheating and loading them), but one can improve the quality of a sensor and one's understanding of its frequency of errors.

The distinction between systematic and random uncertainty is not just philosophical—it is important for decision making (Bier and Lin 2013). If a particular decision is difficult because of a recognized source of epistemic uncertainty, further research or intelligence gathering might be desirable before making a final decision (assuming that time allows and the cost of information gathering is not prohibitive). If a decision is anticipated to be difficult because of aleatory uncertainty, further testing is needed to test the sensors to better qualify the uncertainty, which it may reduce or increase. The primary way to improve the effects of that uncertainty would be to switch to a more reliable or independent detection technology. Still, more or better information *does not necessarily reduce* uncertainties. In fact, it may increase it by uncovering previously unrecognized sources of uncertainty, and that may be critical to a better decision.

C

U.S. Policy-Making Structure for Nuclear War and Nuclear Terrorism

Presidential strategy, decisions, and policy related to nuclear war and nuclear terrorism translate into operational actions and program executions in federal agencies through doctrines, guidelines, and directives. Programs within, and sometimes across, the federal agencies focus on those aspects of the missions that are components of the national strategy. Unclassified details on the organization for managing national strategy related to nuclear war and nuclear terrorism are included, if available.

THE NATIONAL SECURITY COUNCIL

Federal statutes and administration practices, supplemented by congressional oversight, largely define the organizations that U.S. presidents use to guide their decisions and implement policy on a range of topics. Established by the National Security Act of 1947, the National Security Council (NSC) has played a crucial role in advising the President with respect to the integration of domestic, foreign, and military policies relating to the national security, so as to enable the military services and the other departments and agencies of the government to cooperate more effectively in matters involving the national security.

The NSC is led by the National Security Advisor, and its membership includes the U.S. Vice President, members of the President's Cabinet, and heads of other agencies. NSC staff manage the flow of information among the president and the relevant federal agencies, including policy recommendations, strategy, and decisions. The details of the organization and the size of the NSC differ among administrations, but a general hierarchical structure has been maintained over recent administrations (Auserwald 2017). Figure C-1 shows this general structure: the NSC, the Principals Committee (including cabinet members), the Deputies Committee (including cabinet members' deputies), and interagency policy committees[1] (IPCs) (including representatives from relevant federal agencies). Interagency coordination for developing strategy across agencies, as well as implementing policy and decisions, is managed by the IPCs, which are usually organized by region and functional policy topics.

One notable change to the national strategic policy development and implementation was the creation of a Homeland Security Council.[2] Approaches toward this council have varied by administration: the Obama administration combined the NSC and Homeland Security Council into a National Security Staff, and the Trump administration retained both separately but declared the NSC to have authority over both (Bellinger 2021; McInnis and Rollins 2018). Details on Biden's Homeland Security Council have not been announced at the time of this writing.

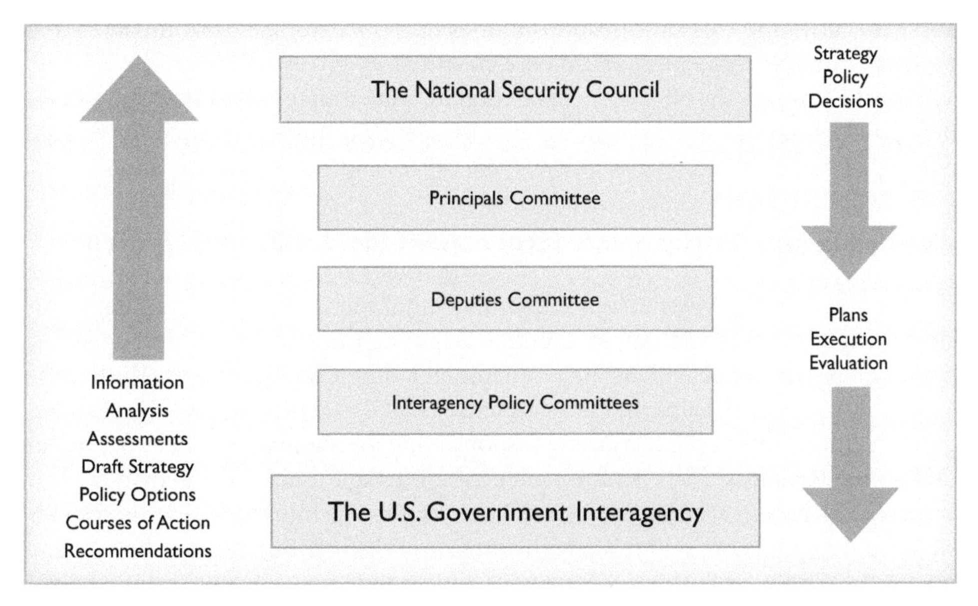

FIGURE C-1 The general organizational structure of the National Security Council.
SOURCE: Joint Special Operations University, 2020, *Special Operations Forces Interagency Reference Guide*, Fourth Edition, U.S. Special Operations Command, MacDill Air Force Base, FL: The JSOU Press, April.

[1] The Obama and Biden administrations have used the term "interagency policy committees," while the G.W. Bush and Trump administrations used "policy coordination committees."

[2] Created by George W. Bush in Executive Order 13228.

TABLE C-1 Presidential Memoranda Defining Structure and Details for the National Security Council

Administration	Presidential Memoranda
G.W. Bush	*National Security Presidential Directive – 1* (Bush 2001)
Obama	*Presidential Policy Directive – 1* (Obama 2009)
Trump	*National Security Presidential Memorandum – 4* (Trump 2017)
Biden	*National Security Memorandum – 2* (Biden 2021b) *National Security Study Memoranda* (Biden 2021a)

PRESIDENTIAL MEMORANDA, DIRECTIVES, AND STRATEGY DOCUMENTS

Presidential policy memoranda can further define and clarify strategy and policy work within the NSC. For example, recent administrations have each issued memoranda defining their NSC structure and details early in their terms (Table C-1). Presidential memoranda on specific topics are issued throughout a presidency and can clarify the roles and responsibilities of the federal agencies involved in a particular policy. Some memoranda are classified.

Acting through the NSC, the president may issue strategic planning documents that drive additional strategies developed by agency leadership, which in turn are developed into operational plans by relevant offices and entities within the agencies.

STRATEGY AND POLICY IMPLEMENTATION: NUCLEAR WAR

Presidential directives define the fundamental role of deterrence strategy, nuclear weapons, and basic employment strategy for the relevant federal agencies, while the National Security Strategy documents offer other guidance. Within the U.S. government, the Department of Defense (DoD) and the National Nuclear Security Administration (NNSA) share responsibility for maintaining the U.S. nuclear deterrence capability. DoD is responsible for ensuring the ability to deliver nuclear weapons, including securely storing fielded weapons, while the NNSA is responsible for designing, surveilling, refurbishing, and dismantling nuclear bombs and warheads. Within DoD, the U.S. Strategic Command manages the operational plans for nuclear employment. The U.S. European Command, which also has responsibility for the day-to-day management of nuclear weapons deployed in Europe, is not part of the U.S. Strategic Command.

To develop their plans, the U.S. Strategic Command relies on guidance from the secretary of defense, who amplifies and implements presidential directives for DoD (U.S. Strategic Command 2020). Documents such as the Nuclear Posture Review (OSD 2018) and National Military Strategy outline broad policy issues. Documents such as the Nuclear Weapons Employment Planning and Posture Guidance, and the Joint Strategic Capabilities Plan further expand on the high-level guidance with more detailed direction and specific objectives.

The directors of the three Department of Energy (DOE) nuclear weapons laboratories—Los Alamos National Laboratory, Lawrence Livermore National Laboratory, and Sandia National Laboratories—are required to complete annual assessments of the safety, reliability, and performance of each weapon type in the nuclear weapons stockpile. In addition, the commander of U.S. Strategic Command provides an assessment of the military effectiveness of the stockpile. These assessments also include a determination as to whether it is necessary to conduct an underground nuclear test to resolve any identified issues. The secretaries of energy and defense are required to submit these reports unaltered to the President, along with any conclusions the secretaries consider appropriate. The letters are an important component of U.S. nuclear deterrence (U.S. House of Representatives 2007).

STRATEGY AND POLICY IMPLEMENTATION: NUCLEAR TERRORISM

Similarly, national strategies for countering nuclear terrorism are developed by the President through the NSC process and are implemented through additional directives and work by the IPCs. Additionally, the President, through NSC staff, oversees federal agency planning, and it is the President who will make the required decisions to activate those plans (JSOU Strategic Studies Department 2013). As noted earlier, interagency coordination is managed by NSC staff and the IPCs, which have important roles of conducting analysis; preparing assessments, strategy drafts, policy options, and courses of action; crafting recommendations; and monitoring the implementation of presidential decisions within their areas of responsibility (JSOU Strategic Studies Department 2013).

AGENCIES INVOLVED IN IMPLEMENTING NUCLEAR COUNTERTERRORISM STRATEGY

Nuclear counterterrorism strategy requires an all-of-government approach. Multiple agencies are involved in implementing the U.S. strategy, as outlined below.

Department of Defense

Since 2016, the Secretary of Defense has tasked the U.S. Special Operations Command (USSOCOM) to coordinate DoD's missions to counter weapons of mass destruction (WMD). This shift away from leadership by the U.S. Strategic Commission Command, which focuses on deterrence, to a USSOCOM-led effort recognizes the latter's more appropriate tools and "activist posture" for nonstate actor threats (Holgate 2018). USSOCOM will prepare *The Global Campaign Plan for the War on Terror* based on strategic documents derived from the Chairman of the Joint Chiefs of Staff's *The National Military Strategy*, which was itself derived from the Secretary of Defense's *National Defense Strategy*, and with input from each geographic combatant commander.

Department of Energy/National Nuclear Security Administration

DOE, through the semiautonomous NNSA, conducts and manages many of its counterproliferation and counterterrorism activities through two main offices: the Office of Defense Nuclear Nonproliferation (DNN) and the Office of Counterterrorism and Counterproliferation (CTCP). DNN has a global mission to prevent terrorists, as well as other countries, from developing nuclear weapons or acquiring weapons-usable material. CTCP works to counter threats of nuclear or radiological material out of regulatory control, a nuclear weapon (out of the owner-state's control), or an improvised nuclear device. Both NNSA offices, as well as other agencies, conduct work countering nuclear terrorism that is managed by and performed at the DOE national laboratories and other industrial facilities.

Department of Homeland Security

The Countering Weapons of Mass Destruction (CWMD) Office within the Department of Homeland Security (DHS) leads the department's efforts to protect the United States from chemical, biological, radiological, nuclear, and health security threats, and in these efforts coordinates with domestic and international partners. CWMD has a mandated role to create and update the Global Nuclear Detection Architecture, which describes a variety of nuclear detection devices and their locations, to help in monitoring for nuclear material or weapons outside of regulatory control. DHS's work on nuclear terrorism risk assessments is shared between DHS Science and Technology, CWMD, and Cybersecurity and Critical Infrastructure Security Agency directorates.

Department of State

The Bureau of International Security and Nonproliferation (ISN) leads work by the Department of State on nuclear security and on treaties related to nuclear security. ISN conducts a range of nuclear security activities, including training and interagency coordination of bilateral and multilateral nonproliferation dialogues. In addition, the Bureau of International Organization Affairs interacts with the

International Atomic Energy Agency and the United Nations on issues related to nuclear security (Holgate 2018).

Department of Justice and the Federal Bureau of Investigation

The U.S. government response to any terrorist-related nuclear activity that may take place on U.S. territory would be led by the Department of Justice and the Federal Bureau of Investigation (FBI) and, through its trained specialists, would provide critical nuclear forensics capacity for use in domestic criminal investigations. Within the FBI, the Weapons of Mass Destruction Directorate interfaces and coordinates globally through Interpol. The FBI also exercises a counter-WMD role with countermeasures before an event, and response planning and exercises postevent.

Intelligence Community

Within the Directorate of National Intelligence, the national intelligence officer for weapons of mass destruction, the National Counterproliferation Center, and the National Counterterrorism Center are directly involved with nuclear security issues. In addition, the Weapons and Counterproliferation Mission Center, within the Central Intelligence Agency (CIA), provides intelligence information and analysis to those involved in relevant programs and policies. Other intelligence agencies have specific nuclear security expertise as it pertains to those missions. In the Biden administration, the director of national intelligence and the director of the CIA participate in the president's NSC meetings in an advisory capacity (Biden 2021b).

DOE's Office of Intelligence and Counterintelligence plays a unique role in the intelligence community because of the unique nuclear expertise resident in the DOE laboratories (e.g., assessing Iran's capability and timeframes to develop nuclear weapons).

U.S. Nuclear Regulatory Commission

The U.S. Nuclear Regulatory Commission (NRC) has, under the Atomic Energy Act of 1954, regulatory authority over spent nuclear fuel, radioisotopes, and certain special nuclear material that could be used in a nuclear terrorism event. The NRC has established security regulations for protection of nuclear material and works with industry partners to ensure compliance. The NRC also has oversight over nuclear power and conducts security evaluations. It works with industry to promote safety/security culture and resilience, reduce sabotage risks, and minimize consequences of incidents.

D

Agendas of Committee Meetings

FEBRUARY 26, 2021

2:00 PM Sponsor and Stakeholder Briefings
Grant Schneider, Professional Staff Member, U.S. House Committee on Armed Services
Leonor Tomero, Deputy Assistant Secretary of Defense for Nuclear and Missile Defense Policy Office of the Under Secretary of Defense for Policy
Rear Admiral Michael Brookes, J2 Intel U.S. Strategic Command
Brigadier General John Weidner, J5 Plans U.S. Strategic Command

3:45 Adjourn Open Session

APRIL 21, 2021

1:15 PM Nuclear War Risk and Possible Scenarios
Martin Hellman, Professor Emeritus, Stanford University

1:45 Nuclear War Risk Analysis Methods and Use
John L. Carozza, Risk of Strategic Deterrence Failure Division Chief, U.S. Strategic Command

Claudio Cioffi-Revilla, University Professor Emeritus, George Mason University

2:45 Adjourn Open Session

APRIL 23, 2021

1:30 PM Nuclear Terrorism Risk Analysis Methods and Use
Steven Streetman, Independent Consultant
Susan Caskey, Global Security Research and Analysis Program, Sandia National Laboratories

2:30 Break

2:40 The Role of Quantitative and Qualitative Methods
George Apostolakis, Professor Emeritus, Massachusetts Institute of Technology

3:10 Public Comment

3:30 Adjourn Open Session and Break

MAY 27, 2021

2:15 PM Jason Reinhardt, National Security Systems Analyst, Sandia National Laboratories

3:00 Henry Willis, Director, Strategy, Policy and Operations Program; Acting Director, Personnel and Resources Program, Homeland Security Operational Analysis Center, RAND Corporation

4:00 Adjourn Open Session

JUNE 18, 2021

12:00 PM Ambassador Ronald Lehman, Counselor to the Director, Lawrence Livermore National Laboratory

12:30 Ambassador Laura Holgate, Senior Fellow, Belfer Center for Science and International Affairs, Harvard University

1:15	Break
1:30	Heather Looney, Senior Advisor, Office of Defense Nuclear Nonproliferation, National Nuclear Security Administration (NNSA)
3:00	Adjourn Open Session

JULY 13, 2021: DATA-GATHERING SESSION (NOT OPEN TO THE PUBLIC)

2:30 PM	Nuclear Nonproliferation Risk Analysis—NNSA Heather Looney, Office of Defense Nuclear Nonproliferation Jeffrey Chamberlin, Office of Material Management and Minimization Zac Palmer, Office of Global Material Security Wayne Mei, Office of Nonproliferation and Arms Control
4:00	Adjourn Data-Gathering Session

E

Committee Member Biographies

WILLIAM C. OSTENDORFF (U.S. Navy—Retired), *Co-Chair*, joined the Naval Academy's Political Science Department as the Class of 1960 distinguished visiting professor in national security in August 2016. Prior to joining the Naval Academy faculty, Captain Ostendorff served as the principal deputy administrator at the National Nuclear Security Administration in the Bush administration (2007–2009) and as a commissioner at the U.S. Nuclear Regulatory Commission in the Obama administration (2010–2016). From 2003 to 2007, he was a member of the staff of the House Armed Services Committee. Captain Ostendorff was an officer in the U.S. Navy from 1976 until he retired in 2002. Entering the Rickover Nuclear Navy, he served on six submarines. During his naval career, he commanded a nuclear attack submarine and a nuclear attack submarine squadron and served as the director of the Division of Mathematics and Science at the U.S. Naval Academy. His military decorations include four awards of the Legion of Merit and numerous unit and campaign awards. Captain Ostendorff earned a bachelor's degree in systems engineering from the U.S. Naval Academy, a law degree from the University of Texas, and a master's degree in international and comparative law from Georgetown University.

M. ELISABETH PATÉ-CORNELL, *Co-Chair*, is the Burt and Deedee McMurtry Professor of Engineering at Stanford University and the founding chair of the Stanford Department of Management Science and Engineering. Her specialty is engineering risk analysis and risk management with applications to complex systems: space, medical, offshore oil platforms, cyber security, national security, etc. Her research has focused first on the optimization of warning systems, including the command-and-control system of nuclear forces and the explicit inclusion of human and organizational factors in the analysis of systems' failure risks. Dr. Paté-Cornell recently received the Ramo medal from the Institute of Electrical and Electronics Engineers for "exceptional achievements in Systems Engineering and Systems Science." Her latest work has focused on the use of game analysis with applications to counterterrorism and cyber security, including artificial intelligence applications to U.S. complex systems that could be targeted by competitors or adversaries. Dr. Paté-Cornell is a member of the U.S. National Academy of Engineering and the NASA Advisory Council and is a distinguished visiting scientist of the Jet Propulsion Laboratory. She was the president of the Society for Risk Analysis (which awarded her the 2010 Ramsey medal) and a member of the President's Foreign Intelligence Advisory Board, as well as several other boards, including those of Aerospace, Inc., and In-Q-Tel. She holds a BS in mathematics and physics (Marseille, France), an engineering degree in applied math/computer science from the Institut Polytechnique de Grenoble, France, and an MS in operations research and a PhD in engineering-economic systems from Stanford University.

DAVID L. BANKS is a professor of the practice of statistics at Duke University. Prior to this, he worked for the National Institute of Standards and Technology, served as the chief statistician of the Department of Transportation, and worked for the U.S. Food and Drug Administration. Dr. Banks was the coordinating editor of the *Journal of the American Statistical Association* and cofounded the journal *Statistics and Public Policy*; he also cofounded the American Statistical Association's (ASA's) Section on National Defense and Homeland Security. He served as the president of the Classification Society and has twice served on the board of directors of the ASA. He is currently the president of the International Society for Business and Industrial Statistics, and a fellow of the ASA and the Institute of Mathematical Statistics. Dr. Banks recently won the ASA's Founders Award. His research areas include models for dynamic networks, dynamic text networks, adversarial risk analysis (i.e., Bayesian behavioral game theory), human rights statistics, agent-based models, forensics, and certain topics in high-dimensional data analysis. Dr. Banks holds a BA in anthropology from the University of Virginia and master's degrees in mathematics and statistics and a PhD in statistics from the Virginia Polytechnic Institute and State University.

VICKI M. BIER is a professor emerita in the Department of Industrial and Systems Engineering and the Department of Engineering Physics at the University of Wisconsin–Madison, where she directed the Center for Human Performance and Risk Analysis, formerly the Center for Human Performance in Complex Systems

(1995–2021). She was recently appointed to the Advisory Committee on Reactor Safeguards of the U.S. Nuclear Regulatory Commission. Dr. Bier has over 40 years of experience in risk analysis for the nuclear power, chemical, petrochemical, and aerospace industries, as well as homeland security and critical-infrastructure protection. Her recent research has focused on applications of risk analysis and related methods to problems of security, critical infrastructure protection, and emergency management. Dr. Bier received the Women's Achievement Award from the American Nuclear Society in 1993 and was elected a fellow of the Society for Risk Analysis in 1996, from which she received the Distinguished Achievement Award in 2007. She is also the past president of the Decision Analysis Society and the editor-in-chief of the society's flagship journal, *Decision Analysis*. Dr. Bier has participated in panels, committees, and subcommittees of the National Academies of Sciences, Engineering, and Medicine, including those dealing with radioactive waste management, a committee to review the Department of Homeland Security's approach to risk analysis, and the Board on Mathematical Sciences and Their Applications (2014–2016). She received a BS in mathematical sciences from Stanford University in 1976 and a PhD in operations research from the Massachusetts Institute of Technology (MIT) in 1983.

MATTHEW G. BUNN is the James R. Schlesinger Professor of the Practice of Energy, National Security, and Foreign Policy at the Harvard Kennedy School. His research interests include nuclear theft and terrorism, nuclear proliferation and measures to control it, the future of nuclear energy and its fuel cycle, and innovation in energy technologies. Before coming to Harvard, Dr. Bunn served as an adviser to the White House Office of Science and Technology Policy, as a study director at the National Academies, and as an editor of *Arms Control Today*. He is the author or coauthor of over 25 books or major technical reports (most recently *Revitalizing Nuclear Security in an Era of Uncertainty*), and over 150 articles in publications ranging from *Science* to *The Washington Post*. Dr. Bunn holds a PhD in technology, management, and policy from MIT.

NANCY J. COOKE is a professor of human systems engineering and the director of the Center for Human and Artificial Intelligence and Robot Teaming at Arizona State University. She is trained as a cognitive psychologist and has researched the assessment of teamwork for nearly 25 years. Dr. Cooke chaired the National Academies' Board on Human Systems Integration from 2012 to 2016 and was a member of the consensus study on safety and security of commercial spent nuclear fuel storage in 2006. She received her BA in psychology from George Mason University in 1981 and her MA and PhD in cognitive psychology from New Mexico State University in 1983 and 1987, respectively.

RAYMOND JEANLOZ is a professor of Earth and planetary science and astronomy at the University of California, Berkeley, and the Annenberg distinguished visiting fellow at the Hoover Institution of Stanford University. In addition to his scientific research on the evolution of planetary interiors and properties of materials at high pressures, he works at the interface between science and policy in areas related to national and international security, resources and the environment, and education. Dr. Jeanloz is a member of JASON, a group that provides technical advice to the U.S. government, and chairs the National Academies' Committee on International Security and Arms Control; he has served on the Secretary of State's International Security Advisory Board and is the past chair of the National Academies' Board on Earth Sciences and Resources. He is an elected fellow of the American Academy of Arts and Sciences, the American Association for the Advancement of Science (AAAS), the American Geophysical Union, the American Physical Society, and the Mineralogical Society of America. Dr. Jeanloz holds a PhD from the California Institute of Technology.

MADHAV V. MARATHE is a distinguished professor in biocomplexity, the division director of the Networks, Simulation Science and Advanced Computing Division at the Biocomplexity Institute and Initiative, and a professor in the Department of Computer Science at the University of Virginia (UVA). His research interests are in network science, computational epidemiology, artificial intelligence, foundations of computing, socially coupled system science, and high-performance computing. Over the past 25 years, he and his colleagues have developed scalable computational methods to study the social, economic, and health impacts of large-scale natural and human-initiated disasters. Those tools and methods have been used in more than 50 case studies to inform and assess various policy questions pertaining to planning and response in the event of such disasters. Before joining UVA, Dr. Marathe held positions at the Virginia Polytechnic Institute and State University and the Los Alamos National Laboratory and was the inaugural George Michael fellow at the Lawrence Livermore National Laboratory. He is a fellow of the AAAS, the Society for Industrial and Applied Mathematics, the Association for Computing Machinery, and the Institute of Electrical and Electronics Engineers. He holds a PhD in computer science from the University at Albany-SUNY.

RICHARD W. MIES is the chief executive officer of The Mies Group, Ltd., a consulting corporation that provides strategic planning and risk assessment advice on international security, energy, and defense issues. A distinguished graduate of the U.S. Naval Academy, Admiral Mies is one of a few flag officers to complete qualification as both a nuclear submariner and naval aviation observer. In his 35-year military career, he has held both U.S. and Allied submarine commands at senior military levels and commanded the U.S. Strategic Command for 4 years prior to retirement in 2002. Following retirement from the Navy, Admiral Mies served as the senior vice president and the deputy group president of Science Applications International Corporation (SAIC), and as the president and the chief executive officer of Hicks and Associates, Inc. (2002–2007), a wholly owned subsidiary of SAIC. He served as the chair of the Department of Defense's Threat Reduction Advisory Committee (2004–2010) and as a member and then the vice chair of the Secretary of Energy Advisory Board. Admiral Mies presently serves as the chair of the Strategic Advisory Group for the U.S. Strategic Command and the co-chair of the Nuclear Energy and National Security Coalition of the Atlantic Council and is a member of the National Academies' Committee on International Security and Arms Control, as well as the Board of Governors of Lawrence Livermore National Laboratory. He also serves on several other research and development-related advisory boards. Admiral Mies completed postgraduate education at Oxford University, the Fletcher School of Law and Diplomacy, and Harvard University, and holds a master's degree in government administration and international relations.

GREGORY S. PARNELL is a professor of practice in industrial engineering in the Department of Industrial Engineering and the director of the MS in operations management (the university's largest graduate program) and the MS in engineering management programs at the University of Arkansas. His research focuses on decision analysis, risk analysis, systems engineering, and resource allocation for defense; intelligence; homeland security; and environmental management. He is a professor emeritus at the U.S. Military Academy at West Point. Previously, Dr. Parnell served as a professor of systems engineering at West Point, a distinguished visiting professor at the U.S. Air Force Academy, an associate professor at Virginia Commonwealth University, and a department head at the Air Force Institute of Technology. He is the former president of the Decision Analysis Society of the Institute for Operations Research and Management Science (INFORMS) and the Military Operations Research Society (MORS). He has also served as the editor of *Military Operations Research*. Dr. Parnell has participated in four committees with the National Academies. He chaired the committees on Methodological Improvements to the Department of Homeland Security's Biological Agent Risk Analysis (2008) and the Review of the Inspection Programs for Offshore Oil and Gas Operations (2021). He was a member of the Committee on Improving Metrics for the Department of Defense Cooperative Threat Reduction Program (2011) and the Committee on Evaluating the Effectiveness of the Global Nuclear Detection Architecture (2013). He is a fellow of the International Committee for Systems Engineering, INFORMS, MORS, and the Society for Decision Professionals. He received his BS in aerospace engineering from the University of Buffalo, his ME in industrial and systems engineering from the University of Florida, his MS in systems management from the University of Southern California, and his PhD in engineering-economic systems from Stanford University. Dr. Parnell is a retired Air Force colonel and a graduate of the Industrial College of the Armed Forces.

SCOTT D. SAGAN is the Caroline S.G. Munro Professor of Political Science, the Mimi and Peter Haas University Fellow in Undergraduate Education, and a senior fellow and the codirector at the Center for International Security and Cooperation in the Freeman Spogli Institute at Stanford University. He also serves as the chair of the American Academy of Arts & Sciences' Committee on International Security Studies. Before joining the Stanford faculty, Dr. Sagan was a lecturer in the Department of Government at Harvard University and served as the special assistant to the director of the Organization of the Joint Chiefs of Staff. He is a scholar of nuclear issues and is the author, among other works, of *Moving Targets: Nuclear Strategy and National Security* (1989); *The Limits of Safety: Organizations, Accidents, and Nuclear Weapons* (1993); and, with coauthor Kenneth N. Waltz, *The Spread of Nuclear Weapons: An Enduring Debate* (2012). In 2017, Dr. Sagan received the International Studies Association's Susan Strange Award, which recognizes the scholar whose "singular intellect, assertiveness, and insight most challenge conventional wisdom and intellectual and organizational complacency" in the international studies community. He received the National Academy of Sciences' William and Katherine Estes Award in 2015 for his work addressing the risks of nuclear weapons use and the causes of nuclear proliferation. Dr. Sagan received his BA from Oberlin College and his PhD in political science from Harvard University.

JAMES SCOURAS is a senior scholar at the Johns Hopkins University Applied Physics Laboratory, where he directs a research program focused on nuclear strategy and global catastrophic risks associated with scientific experimentation. Previously, he was the chief scientist of the Defense Threat Reduction Agency's Advanced Systems and Concepts Office. Dr. Scouras also served as the program director for risk analysis at the Homeland Security Institute, held research positions at the Institute for Defense Analyses and the RAND Corporation, and lectured on nuclear policy in the University of Maryland's General Honors Program. His recent publications include "Nuclear War as a Global Catastrophic Risk" (*Journal of Benefit-Cost Analysis*, 2019) and his edited volume, *On Assessing the Risk of Nuclear War*, published in 2021. Dr. Scouras earned his PhD in 1980 from the University of Maryland and his BS in 1969 from the University of Rochester, both in physics.

PAUL SLOVIC is the president of the research institute Decision Research, which he cofounded with Sarah Lichtenstein and Baruch Fischhoff in 1976. He has been a professor of psychology at the University of Oregon since 1986. Dr. Slovic and his colleagues worldwide have developed methods to describe risk perceptions and measure their impacts on individuals, industry, and society. His recent research examines "psychic numbing" and the failure to respond to global threats from genocide and nuclear war. Dr. Slovic is a past president of the Society for Risk Analysis, from which he received a Distinguished Contribution Award in 1991. In 1993, he received the Distinguished Scientific Contribution Award from the American Psychological Association, and in 1995, he received the Outstanding Contribution to Science Award from the Oregon Academy of Science. Dr. Slovic has received honorary doctorates from the Stockholm School of Economics (1996) and the University of East Anglia (2005). He was elected to the American Academy of Arts & Sciences in 2015 and the National Academy of Sciences in 2016. He received the 2022 Bower Award and Prize, given by The Franklin Institute for foundational and theoretical contributions to the study of decision making. Dr. Slovic has served on numerous committees of the National Academies, including those that produced the reports *Risk Assessment in the Federal Government* (1983) and *Understanding Risk: Informing Decisions in a Democratic Society* (1996). He received his BA from Stanford University and his MA and PhD in psychology from the University of Michigan.

ALYSON G. WILSON is the associate vice chancellor for national security and special research initiatives at North Carolina State University (NC State). She is also a professor in the Department of Statistics and the principal investigator for the Laboratory for Analytic Sciences. Dr. Wilson is a fellow of the ASA and the AAAS. Her research interests include statistical reliability, Bayesian methods, and the application of statistics to problems in defense and national security. Prior to joining NC State, Dr. Wilson was a research staff member at the IDA Science and Technology Policy Institute (2011–2013); an associate professor in the Department of Statistics at Iowa State University (2008–2011); a technical staff member in the Statistical Sciences Group at Los Alamos National Laboratory (1999–2008); and a senior statistician and operations research analyst with Cowboy Programming Resources (1995–1999). In addition to numerous other publications, she has coauthored a book, *Bayesian Reliability*, and coedited two other books, *Statistical Methods in Counterterrorism: Game Theory, Modeling, Syndromic Surveillance, and Biometric Authentication* and *Modern Statistical and Mathematical Methods in Reliability*. Dr. Wilson received her PhD in statistics from Duke University.

NATIONAL ACADEMIES Sciences Engineering Medicine

NATIONAL ACADEMIES PRESS
Washington, DC

Risk Analysis Methods for Nuclear War and Nuclear Terrorism

Committee on Risk Analysis Methods for Nuclear War and Nuclear Terrorism

Board on Mathematical Sciences and Analytics
Division on Engineering and Physical Sciences

Nuclear and Radiation Studies Board
Division on Earth and Life Studies

Committee on International Security and Arms Control
Policy and Global Affairs

Consensus Study Report

NATIONAL ACADEMIES PRESS 500 Fifth Street, NW Washington, DC 20001

This activity was supported by the Department of Defense. Any opinions, findings, conclusions, or recommendations expressed in this publication do not necessarily reflect the views of any organization or agency that provided support for the project.

International Standard Book Number-13: 978-0-309-68998-4
International Standard Book Number-10: 0-309-68998-8
Digital Object Identifier: https://doi.org/10.17226/26609

This publication is available from the National Academies Press, 500 Fifth Street, NW, Keck 360, Washington, DC 20001; (800) 624-6242 or (202) 334-3313; http://www.nap.edu.

Printed in the United States of America.

Suggested citation: National Academies of Sciences, Engineering, and Medicine. 2023. *Risk Analysis Methods for Nuclear War and Nuclear Terrorism*. Washington, DC: The National Academies Press. https://doi.org/10.17226/26609.